With enduring affection, this book is dedicated to Jose Alberto Rodriguez — a guiding light and cherished presence in our lives.

His enduring spirit and the echoes of his warmth remain with us, shaping our journey beyond the realm of sight.

This book is dedicated to my muse, Euridice, to my cherished family and beloved relatives, and to all the friends who have walked with me on this journey. Your love and support have indelibly sculpted the contours of my life.

#AffeStiller #elmonoquieto

Table Of Contents

Prologue

My Journey Through the Food Matrix

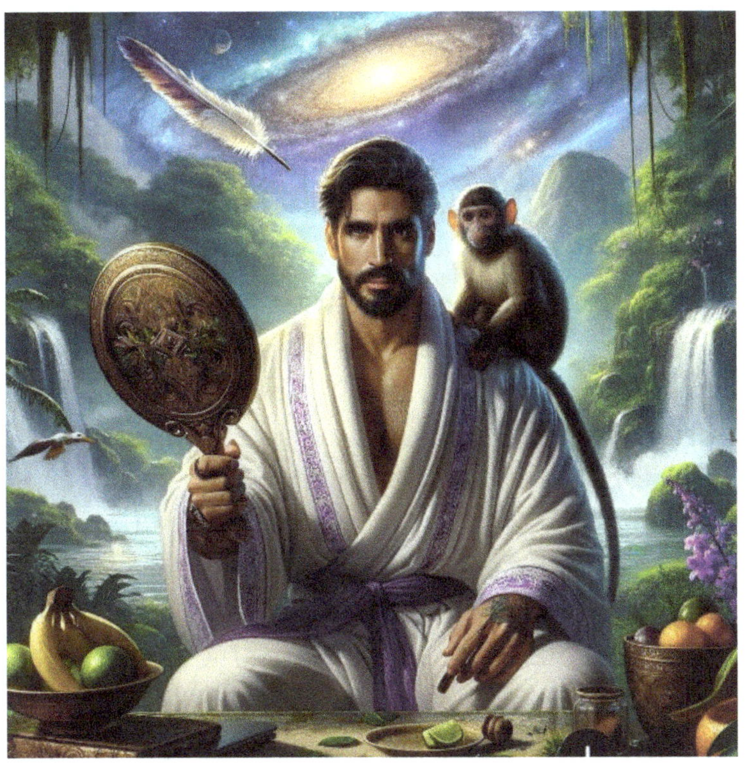

Prologue

The Red Pill Diet

Seven years of delving into the mysteries of longevity and self-care have illuminated my path with a series of illuminations that gradually pieced together the mosaic of what I now know as the "Red Pill Diet." Each revelation, a lantern lighting the way, encouraged a deeper understanding of how we nourish our bodies and souls.

My first illumination emerged from a curiosity about global longevity diets and their cultural signatures. Surprisingly, I found a gap where Mexico's rich dietary heritage should have been. This absence sparked a quest to explore and document the vibrant tapestry of Mexican nutrition. In uncovering the bountiful sources of health within my homeland's cuisine, I discovered a mission: to elevate these findings from local treasures to global knowledge. This mission became the cornerstone of my journey, an imperative to share the wealth of Mexico's diet with the world.

In the fertile ground of this discovery, I nurtured the idea of a healthy food delivery service, born amidst the global pause of the pandemic. This initiative was more than a business; it was a lifeline to connect people with the essence of Mexican longevity through nourishment.

The Red Pill Diet

Drawing from my deep dive into Mexico's dietary wisdom, I next turned my gaze northward, contemplating how to intertwine the richness of Mexican food traditions with the diverse tapestry of American dietary preferences.

This exploration was not merely a business challenge but a cultural journey, seeking harmony between distinct culinary worlds. It became a dance of flavors and nutrition, balancing authenticity with accessibility, guiding me to find a common language in the universal pursuit of health.

This dialogue between cultures brought me face to face with the entrenched norms dictating our food choices. Challenging these conventions, I realized the power of informed decision-making in our diets.

This understanding was a liberation, freeing me from the constraints of societal expectations and allowing me to advocate for a more mindful approach to eating.

It underscored the transformative potential of knowledge, empowering us to redefine our relationship with food.

The Red Pill Diet

Amidst this awakening, I encountered the concept of the Food Matrix, a framework that resonated with my journey's narrative.

Like the Matrix, our dietary choices are often dictated by unseen forces. Using this analogy, I endeavored to demystify the complexities of nutrition and wellness, making the subject approachable and engaging.

This revelation was a key to unlocking the doors of perception, inviting others to see beyond the veil of dietary dogma and embrace a more conscious way of eating.

My path then led me to share my journey and insights with a wider audience, utilizing the visual language of infographics and illustrations.

 This endeavor was not just about imparting knowledge but about connecting on a human level, fostering a community united in the pursuit of longevity.

It was an invitation to embark on a collective journey towards better health, inspired by the shared stories of transformation.

The Red Pill Diet

The penultimate illumination in my quest was the recognition of the power of media—both digital and physical—to promote a lifestyle of conscious longevity and mindful eating.

I envisioned creating platforms that would not only inform but also inspire action and change.

This vision extended beyond individual wellness to encompass a societal shift towards more sustainable and healthful living practices.

It was a call to question the very essence of our dietary choices, making every bite a moment of mindfulness and every sip a reflection of our commitment to health.

 Finally, the journey brought me full circle to the importance of personal health and self-care as the foundation for any meaningful change. I understood that to inspire others, I must first embody the principles of the lifestyle I advocate. This realization was not a conclusion but a new beginning, an invitation to live by example and lead with authenticity.

In closing, the journey through these illuminations culminated in the recognition that longevity remains an elusive goal, not for its complexity but for its simplicity. The "Red Pill Diet" emerges as a guide to embracing this simplicity, offering a blueprint for crafting a personal diet attuned to one's unique needs and aspirations. It is a testament to the power of attention, a call to reclaim autonomy over our health, and a celebration of the richness of our dietary choices.

Through this book, I invite you to join me in this journey, discovering the boundless potential within us to nourish, thrive, and live fully.

Introduction

•Food as transformative information.

In this relentless, fast-moving era where technology is king, we find ourselves amidst a deluge of advice on sculpting the ideal physique and sustaining a healthy weight. Amidst this cacophony, fleeting solutions abound, promising quick wins but seldom grappling with the root causes of our less-than-ideal eating habits. In penning "The Food Matrix" and "The Red Pill Diet," I diverge from the beaten path, treating food not merely as sustenance but as potent, transformative information.

 This tale defies traditional dieting dogmas, an anthem for the synchronicity between our physical form and the food that fuels it. The essence of my message is both straightforward and transformative: cultivating mindfulness around our eating habits can profoundly change how we interact with food, and in turn, it can lay the foundation for a lifetime of health.

The Red Pill Diet

I've uncovered a powerful truth in learning to listen — truly listen — to the whispers and roars of hunger and satisfaction from within. Food is more than sustenance; it's a dialogue with our deepest selves. It's a daily ritual that can either affirm our health or undermine it, and by bringing a mindful presence to each meal, we choose the former.

This narrative is not a fleeting trend. It's a conscious choice to engage with every flavor, every texture, and every aroma, finding the joy in each bite and the signals that guide our intake. For wellness-focused individuals like myself, eating transforms into an act of self-respect, a moment of connection with our inner wisdom.

As we turn the act of eating into a meditative practice. Together, we will chart a course through The Food Matrix, armed with the knowledge that our mindful choices lead us to holistic well-being. This is our revolution: a movement that honors our individuality by nourishing our bodies.

I delve into the psychology of consumption and its far-reaching implications on our well-being. Food, I argue, transcends its basic function of nourishment; it's a dynamic form of information that shapes our physical, mental, and emotional landscapes. Grasping the transformative essence of food empowers us to make enlightened choices that foster health and facilitate weight loss.

Equipped with personal insights, empirical evidence, and practical advice, this book is a reference for wellness seekers eager to cultivate mindful eating habits. It covers a spectrum of strategies—from mindful meal preparation and intuitive eating to recognizing emotional triggers—designed to nurture a harmonious relationship with food.

Moreover, the narrative acknowledges the peculiar hurdles we face: the omnipresence of social media, hectic schedules, and the allure of processed fare. Tailored to fit the millennial way of life, my guidance encourages readers to enact lasting changes, aligning with their wellness objectives.

The Red Pill Diet

Embarking on a path to holistic well-being, I've embraced mindful eating as a cornerstone of my daily practice. It's a practice that transcends the act of eating and delves into the 'how' and the 'why.' This approach has led me to become acutely attuned to the inner workings of my body—its signals for hunger and satiety that are all too easy to neglect in a world bombarded by external influences.

By truly listening to my body's cues, I've tapped into a profound level of self-awareness. Some say it accounts for as much as 80% of our relationship with food. This heightened awareness has enabled me to decipher my body's language, understanding not just the need to eat but the intricate reasons behind my cravings and choices.

This journey isn't just about the physical benefits, although they are plentiful—from smoother digestion and a revved-up metabolism to balanced energy and an uplifted mood. It's about connecting with food on a deeper level, recognizing its journey to my plate, and its impact not just on me, but on the environment. It's about respect for the nourishment provided and the hands that have toiled to produce it.

The Red Pill Diet

Mindful eating isn't confined to the realms of dieting; it's far removed from the constraints of restriction. Instead, it's a liberating lifestyle choice, a skill that I've woven into the fabric of my daily life. Each meal is an opportunity to practice, to grow, and to nourish not just my body but my soul.

In the simplicity of this practice lies its beauty. With every mindful bite, I'm choosing a life of awareness, a life where my food decisions align with my deepest values for health and well-being. This is the essence of The Red Pill Diet—a diet stripped of illusions, focused on the authentic self, and rooted in the mindful appreciation of life's most basic sustenance.

"The Food Matrix" reframes the discourse on weight management and nutrition, underscoring the pivotal role of food as transformative information. By embracing mindful eating, we don't just inch closer to our well-being aspirations; we also cultivate a nourishing bond with food, a legacy that will enrich our lives for years to come.

Decoding Nutrition:

The Singular Disease Theory and the Commodification of Health

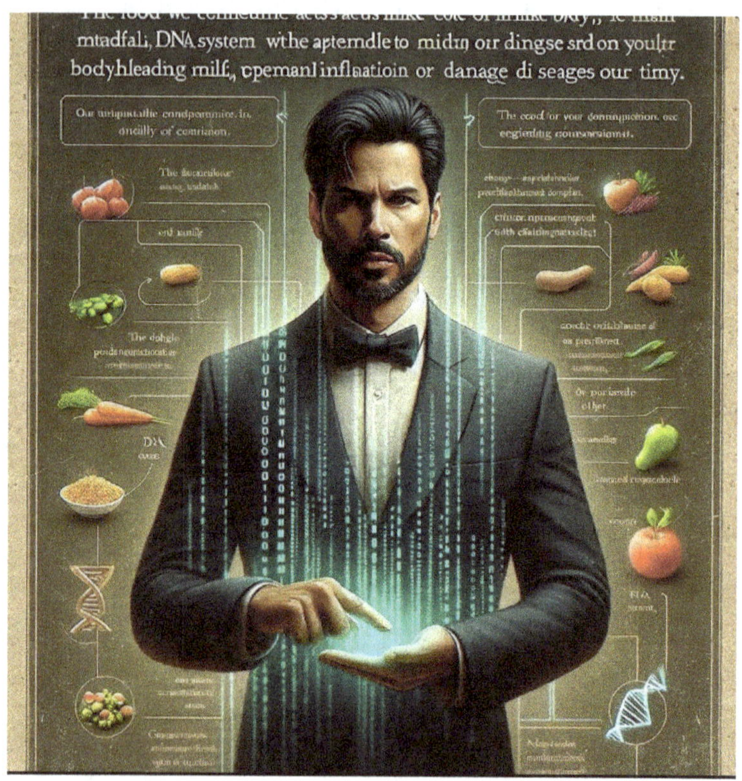

What you consume information (molecules), and your body operates as an editable system. This concept suggests that the food you eat acts like code, which in turn possesses the ability to edit the code (DNA) within each of your cells, thereby enhancing the system or, conversely, infecting it, damaging it, and hacking the system (your body) to become addicted to malicious codes. Just as two individuals are never exactly alike, they also do not consume precisely the same things. This variance leads to each person developing a different type of mild and permanent inflammation that accumulates over time until it morphs into a disease.

In essence, regarding food and nutrition-related illnesses, there is fundamentally one underlying condition—metabolic syndrome. However, this syndrome manifests through various branches, each identified by a different name based on the type of inflammation it causes. This complexity has necessitated a specialization within the medical field, with a focus on addressing the myriad forms of inflammation and bodily harm. Regrettably, the healthcare industry is often influenced by 'the machines,' a metaphor for entities prioritizing profit over health. Instead of concentrating on treating the root causes of inflammation, there's a tendency to commercialize illness, shifting the focus away from holistic healing.

Chapter 1:
What is the Food Matrix

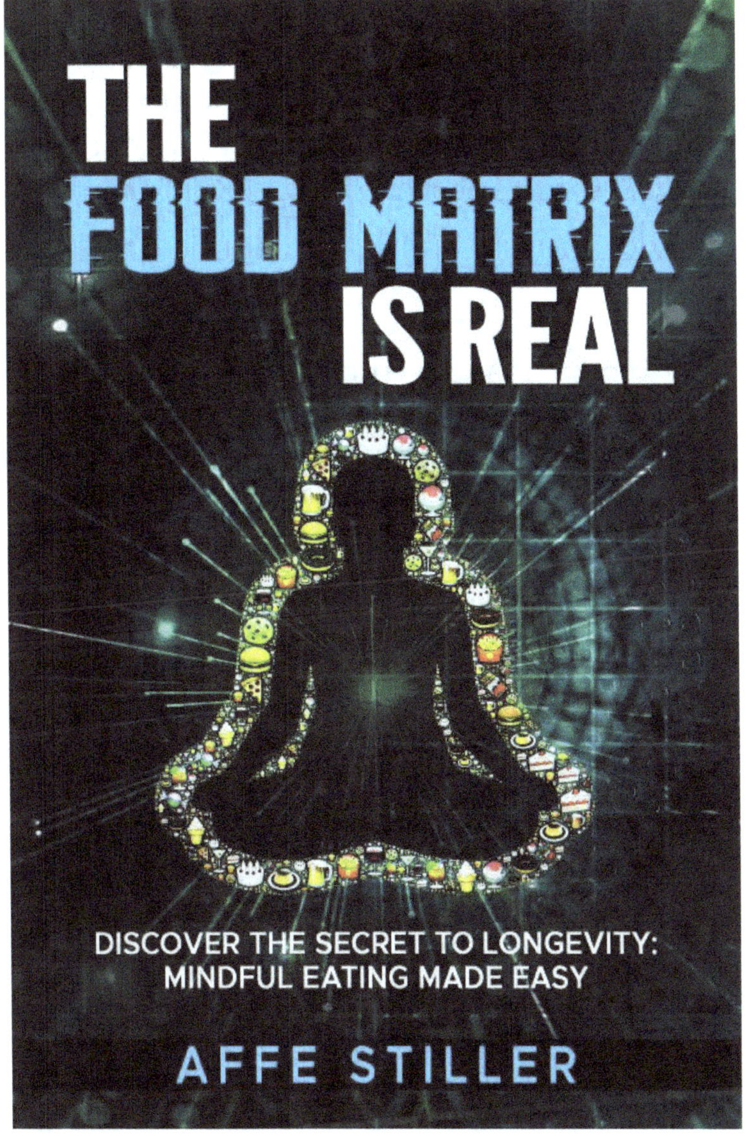

whatisthefoodmatrix.com

· The Food Matrix revealed

My awakening to the realities of The Food Matrix—a construct designed by profit-driven entities to shape our dietary preferences from a young age—has been both enlightening and alarming. This matrix, fueled by the strategic manipulation of sugar, caffeine, salt, and fat, aims to keep us addicted, unknowingly contributing to our own health's detriment.

Recognizing that these choices were never indeed mine was a pivotal moment. Realizing that my preferences could have been engineered from birth by external forces was shocking and liberating. It spurred me to question everything I thought I knew about food and nutrition.

Choosing the Red Pill Diet

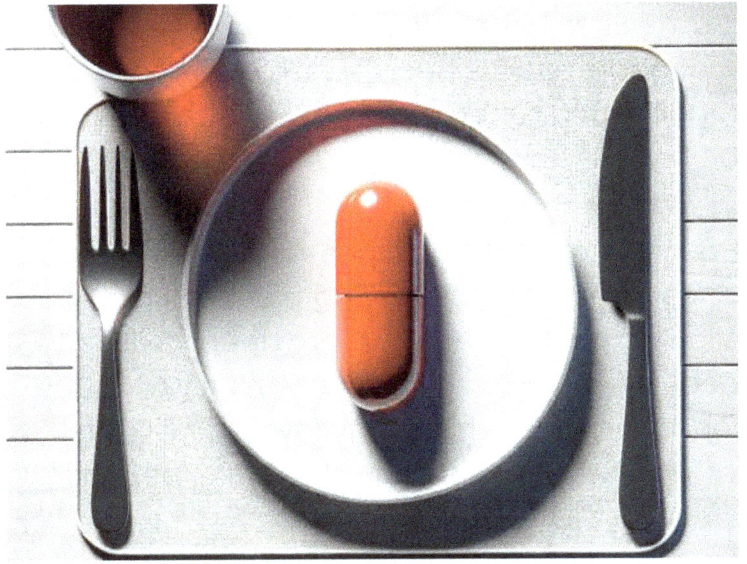

The Red Pill Diet

The decision to adopt what I've come to call The Red Pill Diet was born from a desire to break free from The Food Matrix's grasp. This journey has been about more than just weight management; it's been a path towards regaining autonomy over my health and well-being.

Embracing whole, unprocessed foods and engaging in mindful eating practices has allowed me to connect more deeply with my body's needs. Discovering the true impact of food on my health, energy levels, and overall vitality has been an enlightening experience.

Mindful Eating as Rebellion

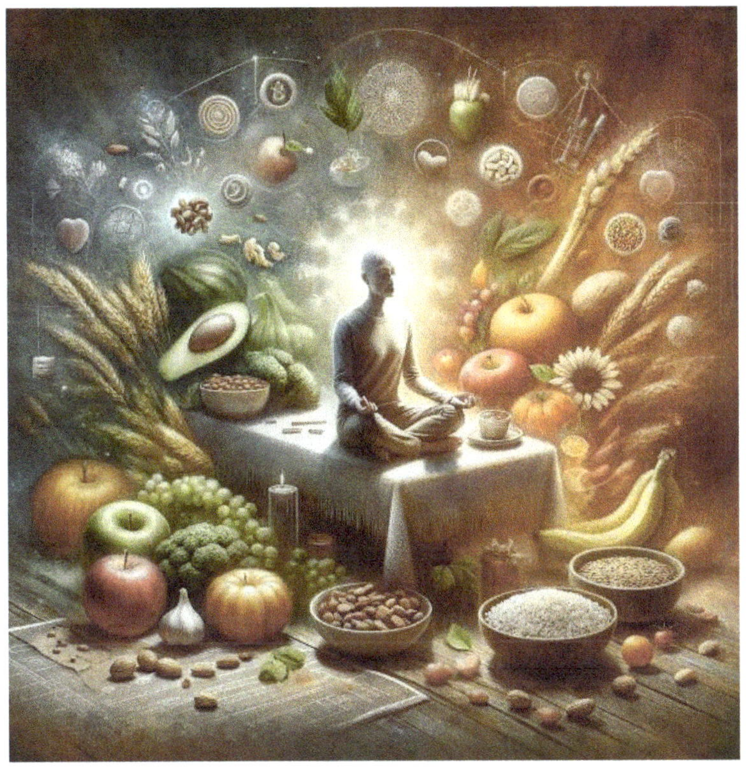

The Red Pill Diet

Mindful eating has become my form of rebellion against The Machines of the food industry. It's a practice that demands presence, awareness, and a commitment to nourishing my body with what it truly needs. This approach has transformed my relationship with food from one of mindless consumption to one of mindful appreciation.

By prioritizing foods that are as close to their natural state as possible and preparing my meals with care, I've found a sustainable way to support not just my health but the health of the planet. This shift toward ethical and sustainable eating practices is a testament to the power of individual choices in driving broader change.

Empowering Others Through Awareness

My journey through the Food Matrix to the Red Pill Diet has been transformative, challenging me to rethink my approach to nutrition and wellness. By sharing my experiences and insights, I hope to empower others to question, explore, and ultimately find their path to holistic well-being.

The fight for a healthier future—a future where we all make informed choices that benefit our bodies and the world—is ongoing. But it's a fight worth engaging in, armed with knowledge, mindfulness, and a steadfast commitment to wellness.

- "Bliss Point: How Additives Manipulate Our Eating Habits

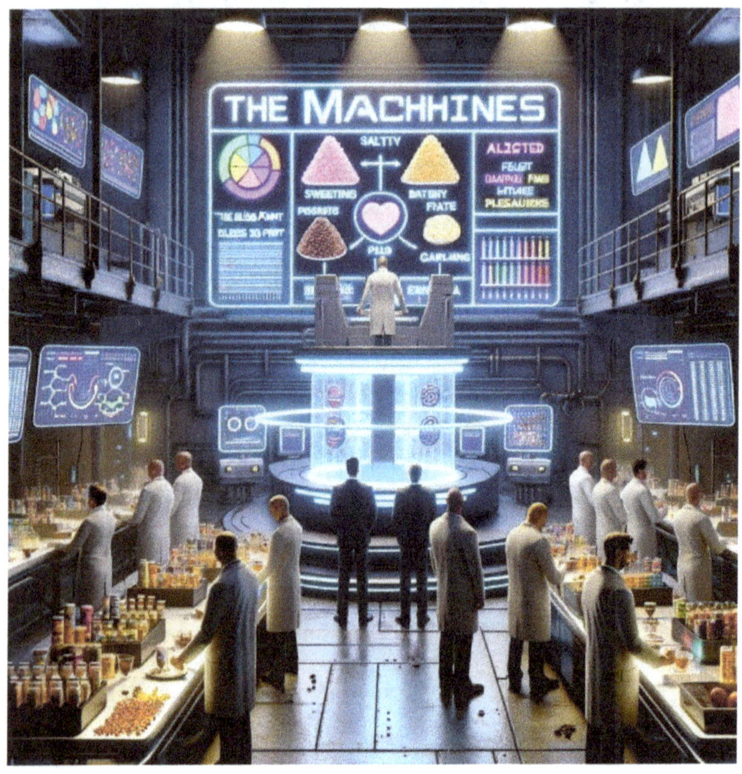

The Red Pill Diet

 The lure of convenience and instant gratification reigns supreme; it's hardly surprising that wellness seekers often find ourselves in a tangle between food choices and nutritional well-being. With its cunning, the food industry has leveraged our innate desires, exploiting our cravings for sugar, caffeine, salt, and fat to their advantage. This narrative delves into the realm of the "bliss point"—a term that encapsulates the exact concoction of ingredients that fires up the maximum pleasure centers in our brains, leading us down a path of overconsumption, weight gain, and unhealthy eating habits.

As we navigate this landscape, it becomes evident that the bliss point isn't just a concept; it's a strategy employed by food scientists who tirelessly seek the ideal balance of sugar, caffeine, salt, and fat, making processed foods nearly irresistible. The realization hits me: these additives aren't sprinkled into our foods by chance. Still, they are meticulously calculated to ensure we return, time and again, often at the expense of our health.

The Red Pill Diet

Take sugar, for example; its presence isn't limited to the obvious culprits like sodas and candies. It lurks in the shadows of many processed items—sauces, condiments, and even bread—contributing to a cascade of health issues from weight gain to inflammation and chronic diseases. The journey toward wellness involves a conscious effort to minimize our intake of these processed temptations, favoring the natural sweetness found in fruits and honey, and reclaiming our health from excessive sugar.

Equally, caffeine, salt, and fats are omnipresent in processed offerings, each with their unique way of ensnaring us into dependency, disrupting our body's natural rhythms, or elevating our risk for chronic conditions. Awareness of these additives and their impact on us is the first step toward a holistic well-being and overall health approach.

By championing whole, unprocessed foods and embracing the art of home cooking, we embark on a quest to dismantle the food industry's influence on our diets. It's about becoming informed consumers, recognizing that our choices can transform our health and dictate the future of food production.

In weaving through the intricacies of the bliss point, this exploration underscores the manipulative tactics of the food industry through additives like sugar, caffeine, salt, and fat. Yet, it also lights the path for wellness seekers to seize control of our dietary choices. By opting for healthier alternatives and practicing mindfulness in our eating habits, we set the stage for a lifestyle marked by sustainable weight management and a deeper, more nourishing connection with our food.

• The illusion of choice in the modern diet.

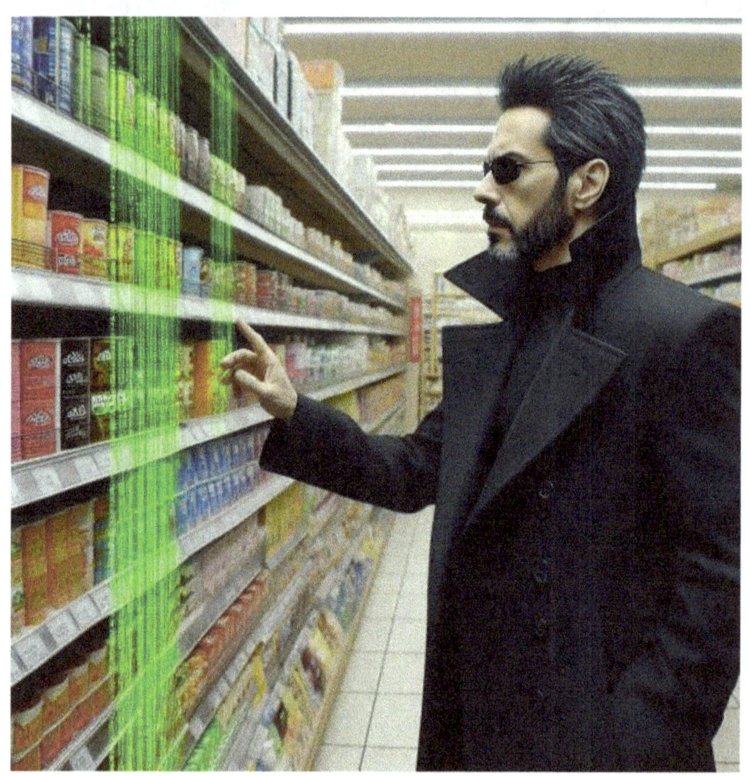

The Red Pill Diet

In this modern era, I find myself navigating through a maze of food choices, like many of my fellow wellness seekers. Supermarket aisles, fast-food chains, and restaurants bombard us with endless options. At first glance, it appears we're spoiled for choice regarding our diets. Yet, upon closer examination, I've realized this perceived abundance of choice is an illusion.

With its clever marketing strategies, the food industry has flooded the market with products all vying for the title of the healthiest option. Low-fat, gluten-free, sugar-free, organic —the labels are endless, each promising a healthier you. But beneath this veneer of choice lies a stark reality: most options are highly processed, packed with additives, and devoid of the nutrients our bodies need.

We're especially vulnerable as wellness seekers caught up in the whirlwind of our fast-paced lives and the allure of convenience. We often find ourselves reaching for those ready-made meals or succumbing to the temptation of fast food, trading our health and well-being for a few extra minutes.

The Red Pill Diet

It's time for a change. It's time to peel back the curtain on this illusion and embrace mindful eating. Mindful eating isn't just about eating slowly or savoring every bite—it's about being present and making conscious, informed decisions about what we eat, understanding the profound impact those choices have on our bodies.

The first step? Educating ourselves on the food industry's sleights of hand—the tricks and tactics designed to lure us into making choices that aren't in our best interest. By learning about the detrimental effects of processed foods and artificial additives, we can see through the façade of choice we've been presented with.

This narrative is more than just a critique; it's a guide. It aims to dissect the deceptive marketing strategies that pervade the food industry and offer practical advice on navigating our modern diet. From decoding food labels to comprehending the implications of various ingredients, it's crafted to empower my fellow wellness seekers with the knowledge to make choices that truly benefit our health.

We can regain control over our diets by confronting the illusion of choice and adopting a more mindful approach to our eating habits. This journey is about more than just shedding pounds; it's about embarking toward a healthier, more nourishing way of life. Through understanding and action, we can transform how we see food, making holistic well-being an aspiration and a reality.

Food as Information: The Code for Health or Disease

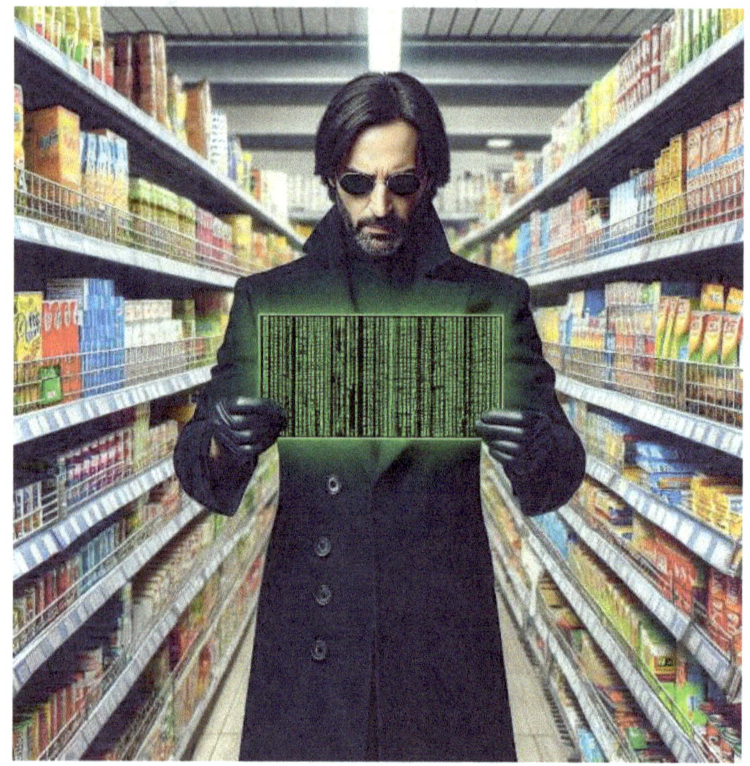

The Red Pill Diet

Diving into the complex world of nutrition, my journey has shifted from viewing food merely as fuel to understanding it as a profound communicator within our bodies. This evolution in perspective has revealed to me that every morsel we consume is a parcel of information, intricately interacting with our biology, influencing our health at the cellular level, and even altering gene expression.

Embracing this knowledge has been transformative. It has allowed me to view my dietary choices through a new lens, recognizing that what I eat is not just about quelling hunger but about consciously curating the messages sent to every cell in my body. This insight has led me to question the prevailing diet trends and the food industry's persuasive marketing, urging me to discern the truth amidst a sea of misinformation.

The Red Pill Diet

This understanding underscores the significance of adopting a holistic approach to what I eat. It's not just the macros that matter but the micros too—the vitamins, minerals, and myriad bioactive compounds that work in concert to support my body's optimal function. It's about embracing a diet that's as varied and vibrant as nature itself, recognizing that our bodies thrive on a diverse spectrum of nutrients.

Moreover, this journey towards nutritional enlightenment has encouraged me to reconnect with the natural world's wisdom, choosing foods that are as close to their earth-grown state as possible. This choice is a commitment to nourishing myself with the full spectrum of life-enhancing nutrients found in unprocessed foods, a testament to the complexity and richness of nature's offerings.

In essence, my path to wellness has been deeply influenced by the realization that food is much more than just sustenance; it's a language, a way of communicating with the deepest parts of ourselves. It's a commitment to providing my body with the best possible information through what I eat, to not just live but to thrive.

Chapter 2:
Breaking the Code

•Unpacking Addictive Additives in Processed Foods

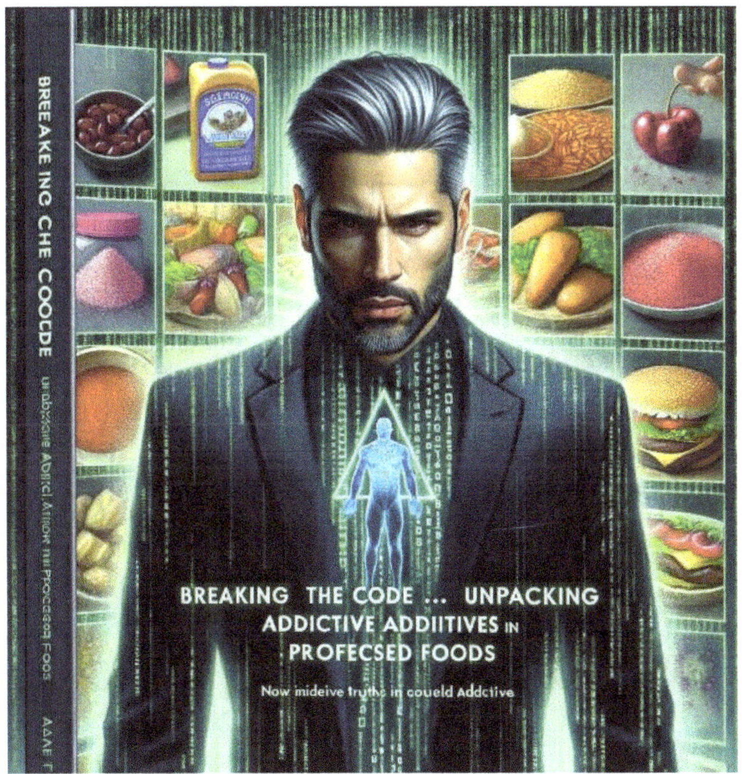

In the quest for holistic well-being, it is essential to delve into the intricacies of our modern diet and its impact on our overall health. One aspect that deserves detailed examination is the presence of addictive substances in processed foods. This subchapter aims to shed light on two substances – High Fructose Corn Syrup (HFCS) and sodium nitrite – that have become ubiquitous in our food supply.

HFCS, a sweetener derived from corn, has found its way into numerous processed foods and beverages. Its excessive consumption has been linked to weight gain, obesity, and an increased risk of developing chronic diseases such as diabetes and heart disease. The main issue with HFCS is its high fructose content, which can disrupt our metabolism and lead to overeating. Moreover, it has an addictive quality that keeps us craving for more, making it difficult to resist the temptation of sugary foods and drinks.

Another concerning substance commonly found in processed meats like hot dogs and bacon is sodium nitrite. It is primarily used as a preservative and gives these products their appealing red color. However, research has shown that sodium nitrite can form harmful compounds called nitrosamines when exposed to high heat during cooking or digestion. These nitrosamines have been linked to an increased risk of developing certain types of cancer, particularly colorectal cancer. Therefore, it is crucial to be mindful of our intake of processed meats and opt for healthier alternatives whenever possible.

Understanding the presence and effects of addictive substances in our food is crucial for wellness seekers seeking holistic well-being and improved nutrition. By being mindful of the foods we consume, we can make informed choices and prioritize our long-term health and well-being. Reading food labels, reducing our consumption of processed foods, and opting for whole, unprocessed alternatives are steps we can take to minimize our exposure to these addictive substances.

•Unplugging from Inherited Eating Habits:
the illusion of free choice.

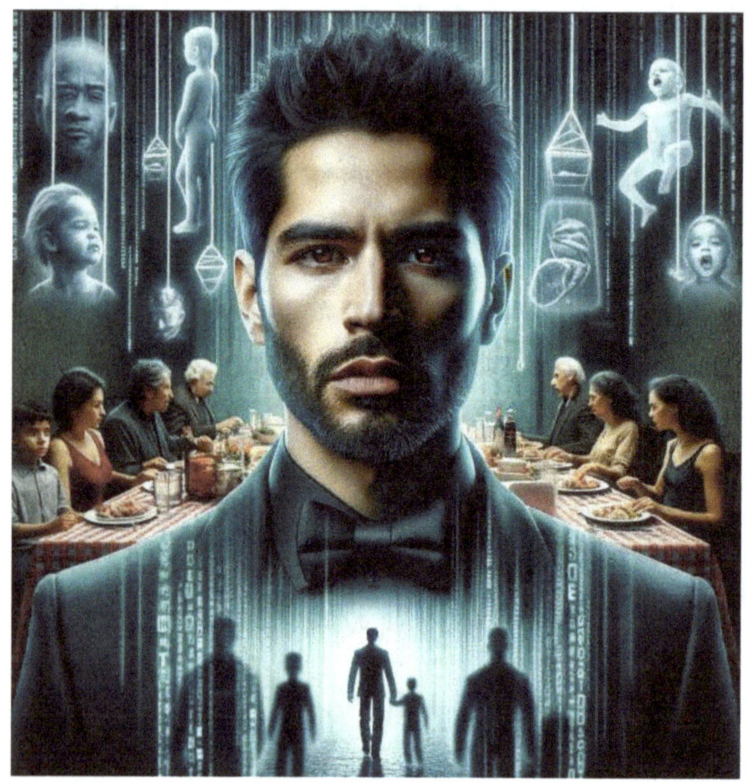

The Red Pill Diet

In this quest for sustainable wellness, I've been compelled to dissect the complexities of our modern diet and its profound implications on our health. In this narrative, my focus zeroes in on a subtle yet pervasive influence: the generational transmission of dietary preferences and the deceptive sense of autonomy we often take pride in. As a health-conscious individual, part of a cohort celebrated for its independence and uniqueness, it's jarring to acknowledge that my eating habits might not be entirely of my own.

Reflecting on my earliest memories, it's clear that the dietary patterns of my family have left an indelible mark on my palate. Whether it was the home-cooked meals that filled our kitchen with warmth or the occasional indulgence in fast food as a treat, these experiences have quietly sculpted my taste preferences and dietary inclinations. This realization challenges the notion of absolute freedom in our food choices, revealing how deeply our family and cultural milieu embed themselves in our subconscious.

The Red Pill Diet

Despite our generation's insistence on autonomy, our culinary preferences are invariably tethered to the environments we were nurtured in. Recognizing this doesn't diminish our capacity for change but highlights the importance of mindfulness in reshaping our dietary habits. Our food choices are not merely about satisfying hunger; they're interwoven with emotions and memories, painting a complex tapestry of comfort, celebration, and, sometimes, sorrow.

The illusion of free choice in our dietary decisions becomes apparent once we acknowledge the profound influence of our upbringing. However, awareness is the first step toward transformation. Through mindful eating, we begin to question the origins of our preferences, exploring the depths of our relationship with food beyond surface-level desires.

As we delve further into this journey, mindfulness emerges as a powerful tool in challenging these ingrained habits, offering a path to consciously curate our diets to align with our health and wellness aspirations. This exploration isn't just about altering our eating patterns; it's a deeper quest for autonomy, allowing us to sever the cords of generational influence and cultivate a more intentional approach to nutrition.

• Unveiling the Food Matrix: Its Impact on Society and Mind

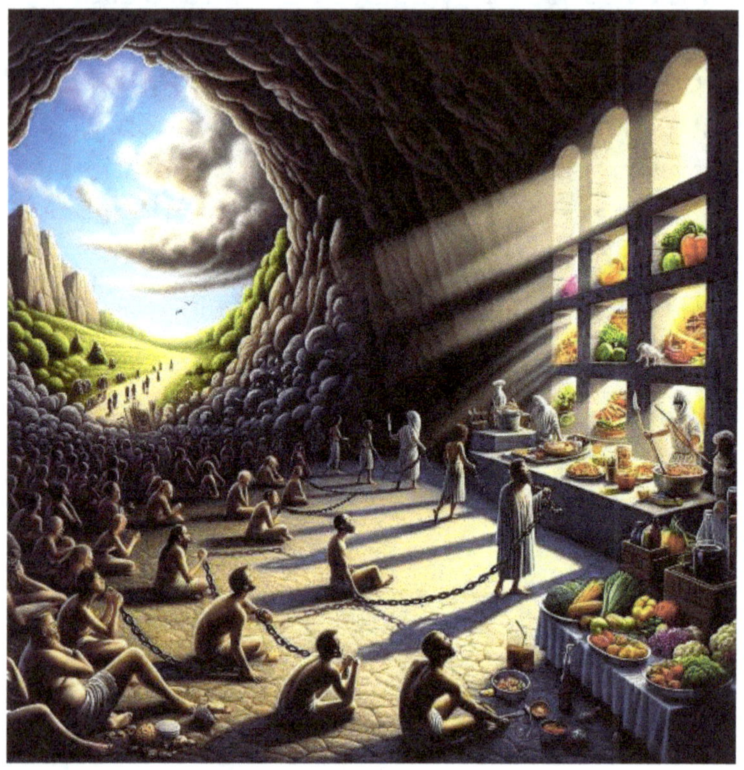

The Red Pill Diet

I've seen how impactful our dietary choices are on our holistic well-being. It's not only about the physical aspect; the ripple effects touch on our social and psychological states. This reflection is about understanding the societal and psychological consequences of what I've begun to see as the Food Matrix, highlighting why mindful eating is crucial for us journeying toward holistic well-being.

The Food Matrix is a term I use to describe the intricate web of influences on our food choices, woven from social, cultural, economic, and psychological threads. Caught in a culture that idolizes convenience and instant gratification, health-conscious individuals like us often find ourselves ensnared, leading to choices that are less than ideal for our health.

Looking through a societal lens, the Food Matrix has fueled a surge in fast food chains and processed food production, encouraging sedentary lifestyles. Our inclination toward convenience means we often reach for foods high in calories but low in nutritional value, sparking a health crisis among health-aware individuals.

Psychologically, the impact is profound. The relentless stream of advertisements, the influence of social media, and the weight of societal expectations forge unrealistic beauty and body image standards. This pressure can lead to dissatisfaction, diminished self-esteem, and unhealthy eating patterns.

Acknowledging the societal and psychological influences of the Food Matrix is the first step in reclaiming our health. Mindful eating serves as a guiding light, leading us toward full presence and making choices that are conscious and in tune with our bodies' signals of hunger and satisfaction.

Embracing mindful eating is liberating. It means breaking away from the Food Matrix's grip, reconnecting with our bodies, and making informed choices supporting physical and psychological nourishment. This path emphasizes the value of whole, nutrient-rich foods, regular physical activity, and a positive food relationship.

The Food Matrix's societal and psychological influences significantly impact those of us striving for holistic well-being. By understanding and confronting these influences, health-minded individuals can regain control over their health, making mindful choices that enhance our overall well-being. Mindful eating isn't just a practice; it's a powerful tool to navigate the complexities of the Food Matrix, leading to a healthier lifestyle and, ultimately, holistic well-being.

Chapter 3: The Red Pill Diet

•Unplugging from the Food Matrix: A Practical Guide

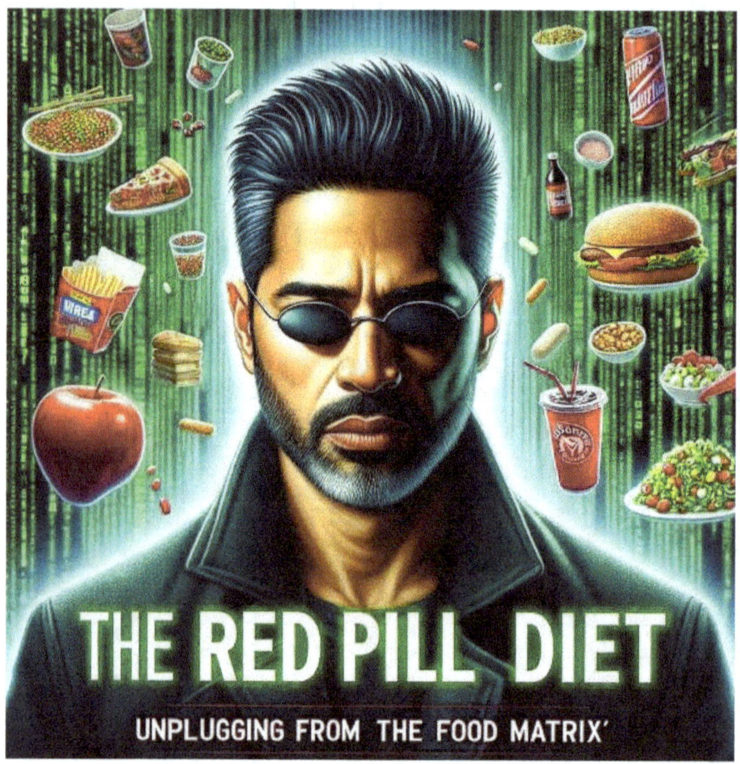

The Red Pill Diet

In this era where life zips by, it's all too easy to slip into a pattern of eating without thought, caught in the tangle of the "Food Matrix." As a wellness enthusiast, this phenomenon hits close to home, with the onslaught of advertisements, social media trends, and the latest diet fads clouding our food choices. But for those of us aiming for holistic well-being, stepping away from this matrix and adopting a mindful approach to eating is vital. Here's how to do it with intention and care:

1. **Challenge Advertising's Lure:** Advertisements wield the power to shape our cravings and desires, often steering us away from our wellness goals. By critically analyzing food marketing and its claims, we can start to see beyond the allure, distinguishing true nutritional value from mere hype.

2. **Listen to Your Body:** The essence of mindful eating lies in syncing with our body's hunger and satiety cues. It's about eating when truly hungry, not just when bored or tempted by the Food Matrix's siren song. Honoring our body's needs leads us down a path of genuine nourishment.

3. **Reduce Food Media Consumption:** The constant barrage of food imagery and discussions can amplify cravings and lead us toward less healthy choices. By limiting our interaction with food-centric media, we surround ourselves with positivity that echoes our holistic wellness aspirations.

4. **Embrace Whole Foods:** The Food Matrix often glorifies processed convenience over nutrition. Shifting our focus to whole, unprocessed foods enriches our diet with essential nutrients, supporting longevity and overall health.

5. **Cultivate Mindful Eating Practices:** Eating slowly, savoring each bite, and appreciating the sensory experiences of food can transform mealtime from a mindless act to a source of joy and satisfaction. It's about creating a serene space free from distractions, allowing us to fully engage with the act of nourishing ourselves.

• The Power of Whole Foods:
The basis of "The Red Pill Diet."

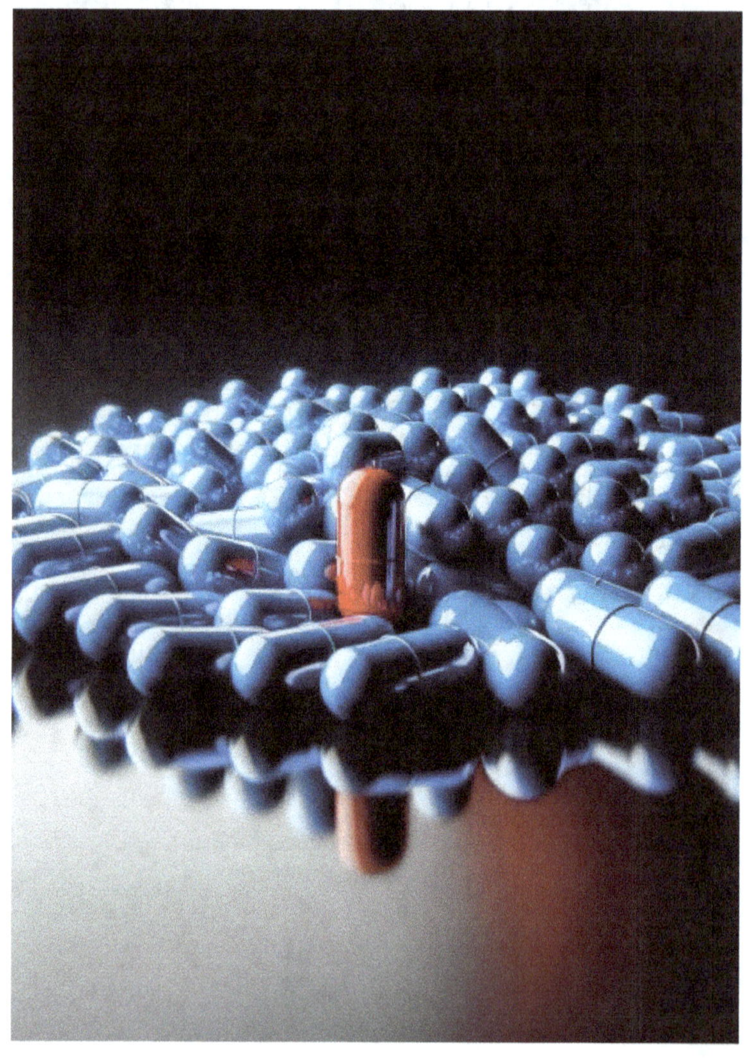

The Red Pill Diet

Adopting these strategies to unplug the Food Matrix empowers us to reclaim our eating habits, setting the stage for holistic well-being. It's about choosing mindfulness and intentionality in our dietary decisions, nourishing both body and soul. Unplug from dietary illusion and open your mind to the power of informed choices.

In this whirlwind of a journey toward true well-being, it's all too easy to get ensnared by the allure of the Food Matrix—the endless stream of fad diets and miracle foods that promise quick fixes but leave us lost in a maze of nutritional confusion. Yet, as I've ventured deeper into the Food Matrix, I've discovered the core of genuine nutrition, unlocking the secrets to a life filled with vitality and nourishment.

At the heart of this revelation is the simple yet profound truth: whole foods, in their least processed forms, are the keystones of our diet. These natural treasures, brimming with essential nutrients, fiber, and phytochemicals, are the building blocks for optimal health, shielding us from chronic illnesses and elevating our physical and mental well-being.

The Red Pill Diet

Embracing the Red Pill Diet, as I've come to know and share within these pages, means making whole foods the cornerstone of our eating habits. This journey has taught me the unparalleled benefits of whole foods—they're not just food but medicine for our bodies and souls. From fostering a thriving gut microbiome, essential for digestion and immunity, to loading us with energy-boosting vitamins, minerals, and antioxidants, whole foods are our allies in achieving and maintaining peak vitality.

But the Red Pill Diet is more than a pathway to personal health; it's a commitment to the health of our planet. Choosing whole foods aligns us with sustainable, ethical eating practices that benefit us and our environment. This choice supports a lower carbon footprint, reduces the need for excessive packaging, and champions local farmers and eco-friendly agriculture.

The Red Pill Diet

In the rhythm of today's life, where fast food and convenience meals often overshadow the essence of nourishment, forging a healthy relationship with food becomes not just a goal but a necessity for wellness-focused individuals like us. This narrative delves into how a blend of passion and dedication can redefine our approach to eating well, highlighting the transformative journey toward holistic well-being.

• Passion and Devotion: Cultivating a healthy relationship with food.

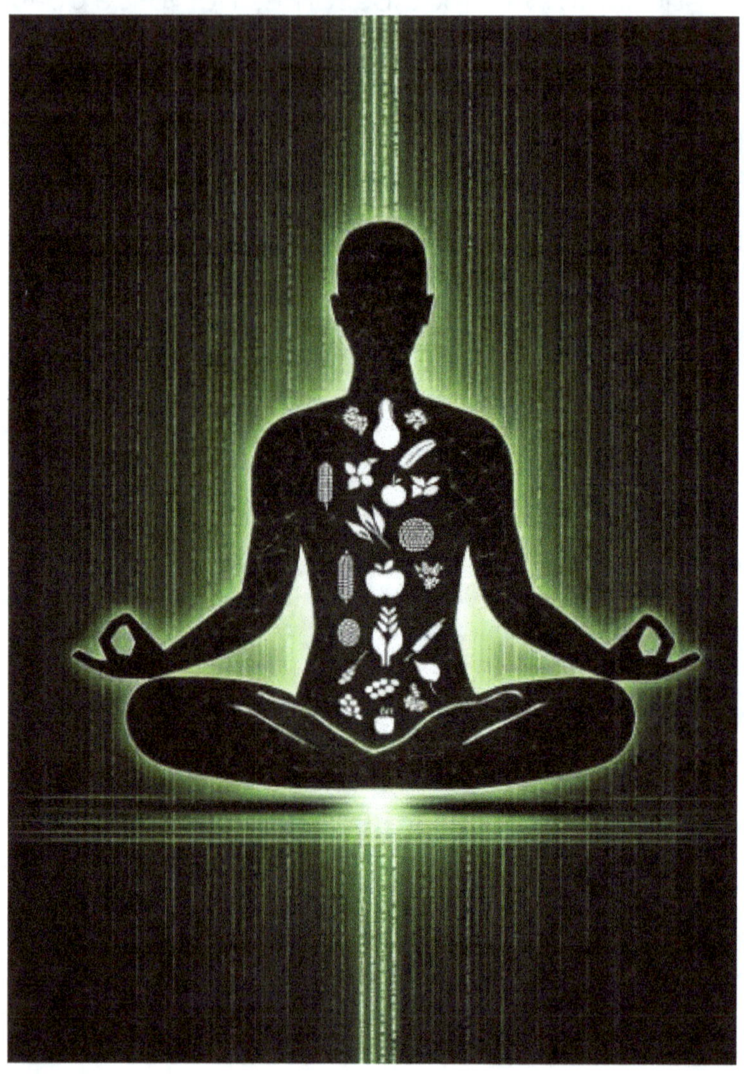

Fostering a Passion for Wholesome Eating: My journey into the world of nutrition has taught me that passion for food transcends mere eating. It's about embracing the rich mosaic of flavors, textures, and each ingredient's nutritional value. This passion has propelled me to venture beyond the mundane, exploring vibrant recipes, integrating fresh ingredients, and connecting deeply with every meal I consume.

The Essence of Devotion to Health: Devotion in this context signifies a steadfast commitment to mindful dietary choices. It's about arming myself with knowledge on nutrition, understanding the pivotal role of various food groups, and aligning my choices with my wellness aspirations. This dedication is the cornerstone of my journey toward sustained well-being.

Prioritizing Quality in Nourishment: My mantra has been to focus on the quality of the foods I eat rather than the quantity. Opting for whole, minimally processed foods has opened up a world of rich, essential nutrients, cutting down on unnecessary additives and empty calories. This shift has enhanced the enjoyment of natural flavors and led to a more gratifying and healthful eating experience.

Embracing Mindful Eating: Mindful eating has revolutionized my relationship with food. Being fully present, savoring each morsel, and tuning into my body's cues have fostered a profound appreciation for the nourishment provided by my meals. This practice has encouraged gratitude, curbed overindulgence, and enriched my eating experience.

Joy in the Ritual of Cooking: Discovering the joy in preparing meals has been a pivotal aspect of my passion and dedication to healthy eating. Cooking has become an expressive journey to channel love and care for myself and those around me. By cooking wholesome meals from scratch, I underscore my commitment to health, crafting an environment ripe for nurturing healthy eating habits.

Embarking on this path demands more than just fleeting interest; it requires a deep-seated passion and unwavering dedication to health. Through embracing the joy of food, prioritizing quality, practicing mindfulness at the dining table, and reveling in the act of cooking, I've found a sustainable route to nourishing both body and soul.

• Mindful Eating:
Keys to Informed Dietary Choices

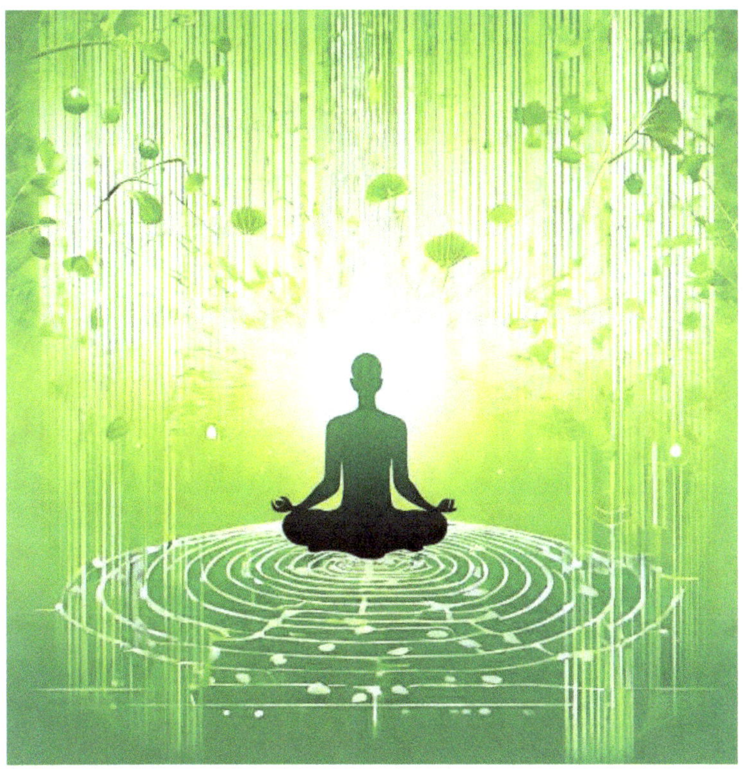

The Red Pill Diet

Navigating today's fast-paced lifestyle, the quest for holistic well-being amidst a sea of fad diets and conflicting nutritional advice is a challenge many of us face. As a health-aware individual, I've discovered the importance of establishing strategies not just for temporary gains but for lasting health and happiness. This journey has led me to share some strategies that have helped me make enlightened dietary choices and embrace a more mindful way of eating.

1. **Educate Yourself on Nutrition:** The digital age, with its influencers and wellness gurus, often leads us down a path of misinformation. I took it upon myself to learn the fundamentals of nutrition—understanding macronutrients, micronutrients, and the truth behind carbs, fats, and sugars. This knowledge has empowered me to sift through myths and make choices that truly benefit my health.

2. **Embrace Mindful Eating:** Mindfulness has been a game-changer for me. It's about being fully present with each meal, appreciating the flavors, and listening to my body's signals. This approach has helped me manage portion sizes, curb emotional eating, and cultivate a positive relationship with food.

3. **Plan Ahead:** I've found that meal planning and prepping are invaluable. By deciding my meals in advance, I ensure that I always have healthy and nourishing options at hand, preventing last-minute, less-than-ideal food choices.

4. **Prioritize Whole Foods:** Steering my diet toward whole, unprocessed foods has been transformative. Fruits, vegetables, lean proteins, and whole grains are now staples of my diet, providing me with the energy and nutrients I need to thrive.
5. **Find Your Tribe:** Journeying toward better health is more rewarding and sustainable with a support system. Whether it's online communities, fitness classes, or a group of friends, sharing goals and experiences with like-minded individuals keeps me motivated and accountable.

By adopting these strategies, I've been able to navigate through the noise of the Food Matrix, making informed choices that align with my pursuit of holistic well-being and mindful longevity. It's a reminder that achieving health is not about restrictive diets but about fostering a balanced, mindful lifestyle.

When walking, walk. When eating, eat. - a Zen proverb.

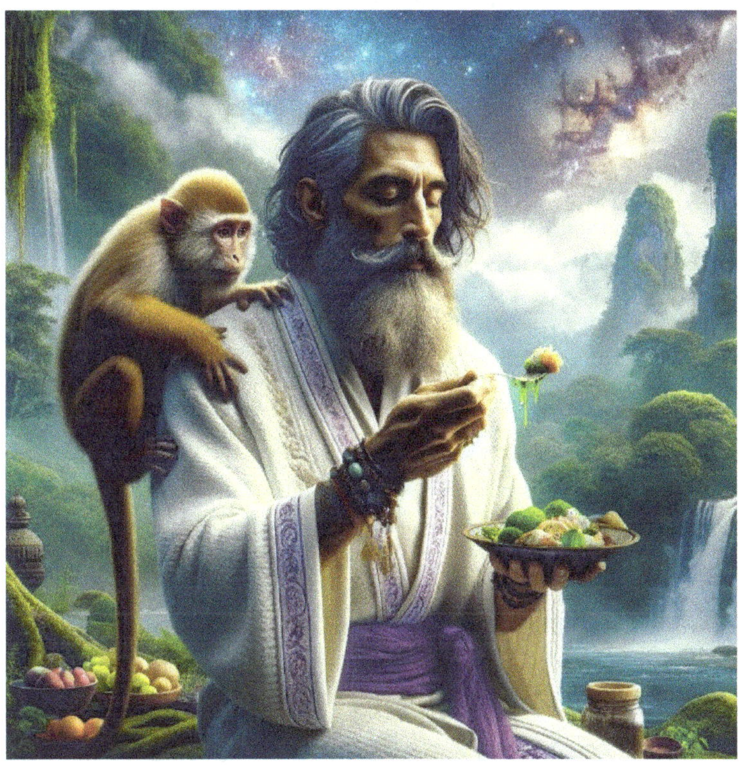

This wisdom has illuminated my path, teaching me the art of mindfulness, especially in nourishment and movement. As someone deeply immersed in the quest for health and vitality, I've realized the transformative power of being fully present in each moment.

The Red Pill Diet

In the complex and sometimes bewildering world of nutrition, mindfulness stands out not merely as a habit but as a shining light of clarity. The habit of juggling tasks—even during meals or while moving from one place to another—disconnects us from the act of truly nourishing our bodies. It's easy to ignore the signals our bodies send us, like the gentle nudge when we're full or the subtle cues of what our bodies genuinely crave for nourishment.

By embracing the essence of the Zen proverb, I've learned to give my undivided attention to the experience of eating. Mindful eating has taught me to appreciate my food's flavors, textures, and aromas. It's about savoring each bite, chewing thoughtfully, and honoring my body's signals. This approach has enriched my culinary experiences and guided me toward making more conscious, healthful choices.

Similarly, applying mindfulness to walking has opened up a world of introspection and connection. Instead of being lost in thought or distracted by my phone, I've found joy in simply walking, feeling the earth beneath my feet, and breathing in sync with my steps. This practice has grounded me and enriched my physical well-being, offering stress relief and a deepened sense of peace.

By integrating the wisdom of the Zen proverb into my life, I've transformed my approach to eating and moving. It's not just about what we eat or how much we move, but the quality of attention we bring to these fundamental aspects of living. Mindful eating and walking have become cornerstones of my path to wellness, guiding me toward more intentional, healthful living.

Recognizing and Overcoming Emotional Eating

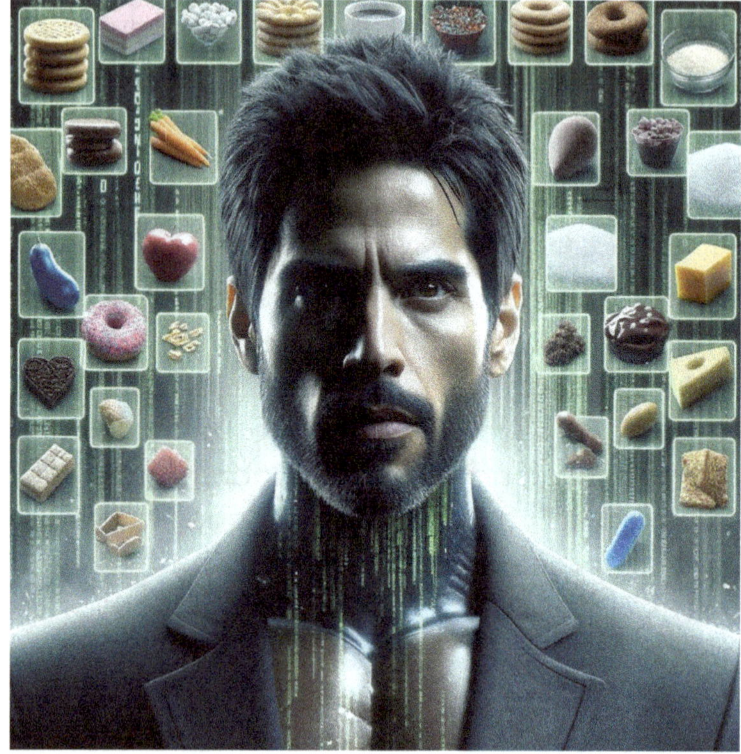

Emotional eating, or reaching for comfort through our meals, has been a personal challenge and a common struggle among those of us committed to wellness. This chapter of my journey delves into understanding emotional eating, facing its consequences, and finding strategies to navigate away from its grasp.

Identifying Emotional Eating: My first realization was acknowledging when I was eating for reasons other than hunger. Was it stress, sadness, or boredom driving me to the kitchen? Recognizing the pattern of seeking out sweets or salty snacks as emotional relief was a turning point. Understanding these triggers was crucial in beginning to untangle myself from emotional eating's hold.

Facing the Consequences: The ramifications of emotional eating stretched beyond just immediate guilt. Over time, it contributed to unwanted weight gain and heightened the risk of chronic health issues, casting a shadow on my mental well-being. This realization— that emotional eating was a temporary fix with lasting consequences—motivated me to seek healthier coping mechanisms.

Building New Coping Mechanisms: Finding joy and relief outside the pantry became my mission. Whether it was a walk in nature, practicing mindfulness, or diving into a creative project, these activities offered genuine solace without the side effects of emotional eating. Cultivating a network of support, where open conversations about struggles and victories could take place, also proved invaluable.

Cultivating a Mindful Relationship with Food: Embracing mindful eating marked a significant shift in my relationship with food. Learning to listen to my body's true hunger and fullness signals helped differentiate physical need from emotional craving. Viewing food as nourishment rather than an emotional crutch allowed me to make choices that aligned with my wellness goals.

Building a Positive Body Image

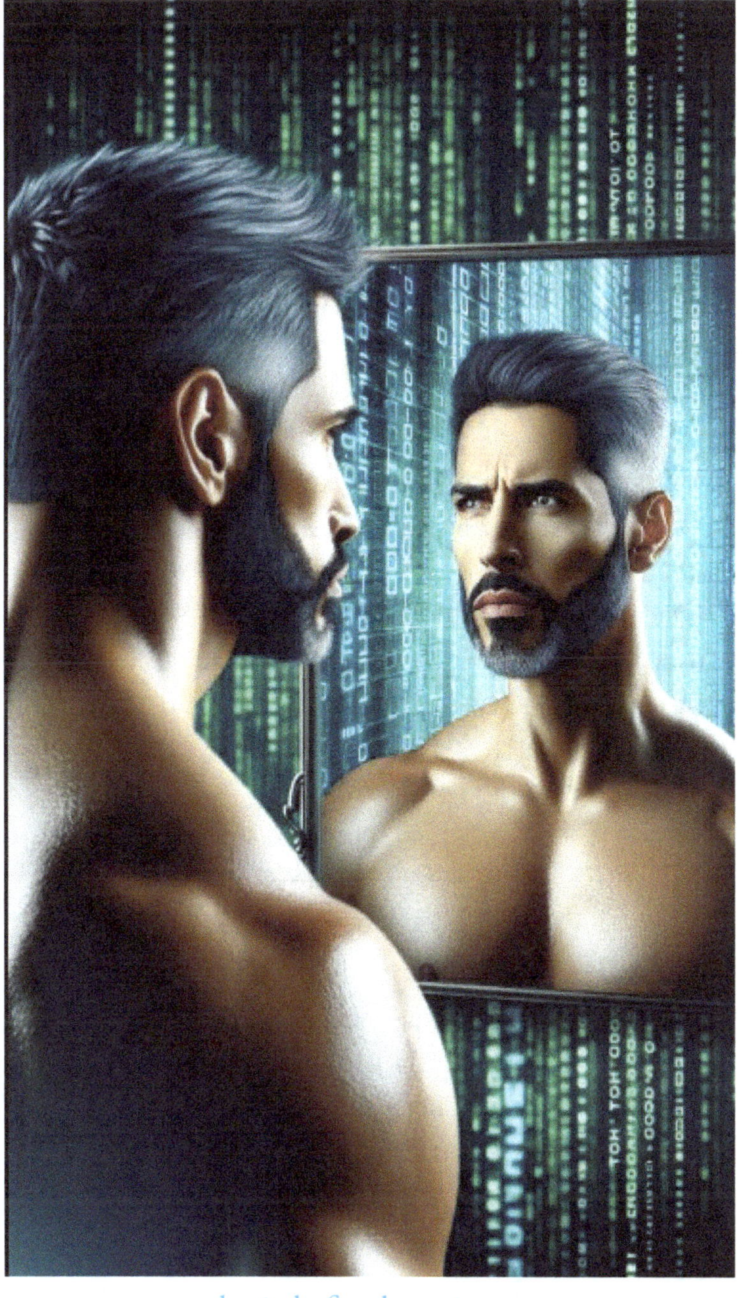

The Red Pill Diet

In my journey toward holistic well-being, I've encountered the challenge of navigating through society's narrow definitions of beauty and health. It's a path that's led me to understand the profound importance of fostering a positive body image. This chapter of my life is a testament to the belief that wellness transcends scales and measurements—it's about embracing our unique bodies and cherishing them for their strength and vitality.

Embracing Our Uniqueness: I've learned to celebrate my body's individuality, recognizing that true beauty lies in diversity. This realization came from understanding that the images we often compare ourselves to are not only unrealistic but also fail to capture the essence of real beauty. My body is a unique vessel that carries me through life, and it deserves love and respect.

Nourishment Over Restriction: Shifting my focus from restrictive eating to nourishing my body was a pivotal moment. I discovered that a healthy relationship with food is not about limiting myself but about providing my body with the nutrients it needs to thrive. It's a mindset shift from dieting to nourishing, which has allowed me to connect with my body on a deeper level.

Cultivating a Supportive Environment: I took steps to curate my surroundings, especially my social media, to reflect positivity and body diversity. This meant unfollowing accounts that fueled negative self-comparison and seeking out communities that uplift and support body positivity. Surrounding myself with messages of self-love and acceptance has been crucial in nurturing a positive body image.

Celebrating Movement: I've also redefined my relationship with exercise. Instead of viewing it as a task or punishment, I now see physical activity as a celebration of what my body can do. Finding joy in movement, whether it's yoga, dancing, or biking, has improved my physical and mental health.

This journey to building a positive body image is deeply intertwined with my quest for holistic well-being. It's about looking beyond societal pressures and embracing our bodies for the incredible work they do every day.

The Power of Mindful Eating

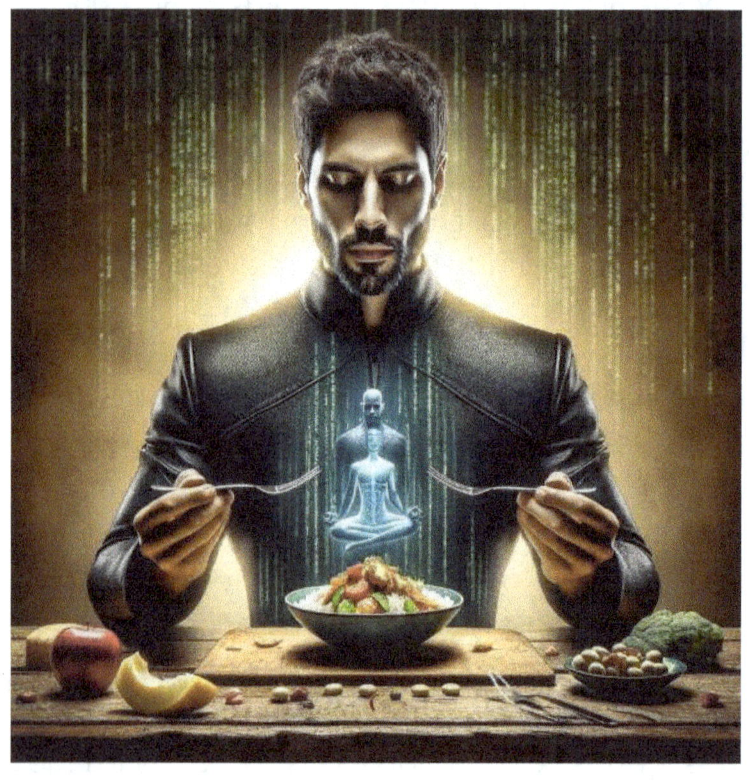

The Red Pill Diet

Surrounded by the allure of quick fixes and instant gratification, I've learned that a more intentional approach to nourishment could fundamentally change my relationship with food and foster profound health improvements.

Mindful eating, to me, is an art—the art of being fully present with every bite, savoring the flavors, and listening intently to my body's cues. It's a practice that transcends the act of eating; it's about cultivating a moment of connection with myself and the nourishment I choose. This practice has opened my eyes to the true experience of eating, allowing me to appreciate the journey of each meal from the plate to my palate and, ultimately, to my soul.

This approach has been a cornerstone in managing my weight more mindfully. Slowing down and truly engaging with my meals has taught me to recognize when I'm genuinely satisfied, reducing the impulse to overindulge. More than that, it's helped me identify the emotional triggers—stress, boredom, sadness —that often led me to seek comfort in food, enabling me to address these feelings more healthily.

The Red Pill Diet

Beyond weight, mindful eating has enhanced my digestion. Taking time to chew and enjoy my food thoroughly has made meals more pleasurable and optimized my body's ability to digest and absorb nutrients effectively. This attentiveness during eating has also minimized digestive discomfort, transforming mealtime into an opportunity for nourishment and healing.

But the most profound impact of mindful eating has been on my mental and emotional well-being. This practice has shifted my perspective on food from one of guilt and restriction to one of gratitude and fulfillment. It's allowed me to break free from the cycle of emotional eating, replacing it with a nourishing ritual that supports my overall happiness and stress relief.

The essence of mindful eating is not just in choosing what to eat but in changing how we eat. For me and fellow wellness seekers, it's a pathway to a deeper understanding of our bodies and needs, guiding us toward a balanced, healthful existence. It's a gentle reminder that in the act of eating, like in life, being fully present can unlock a world of joy and discovery.

Chapter 4:
Designing Your Personal Red Pill Diet

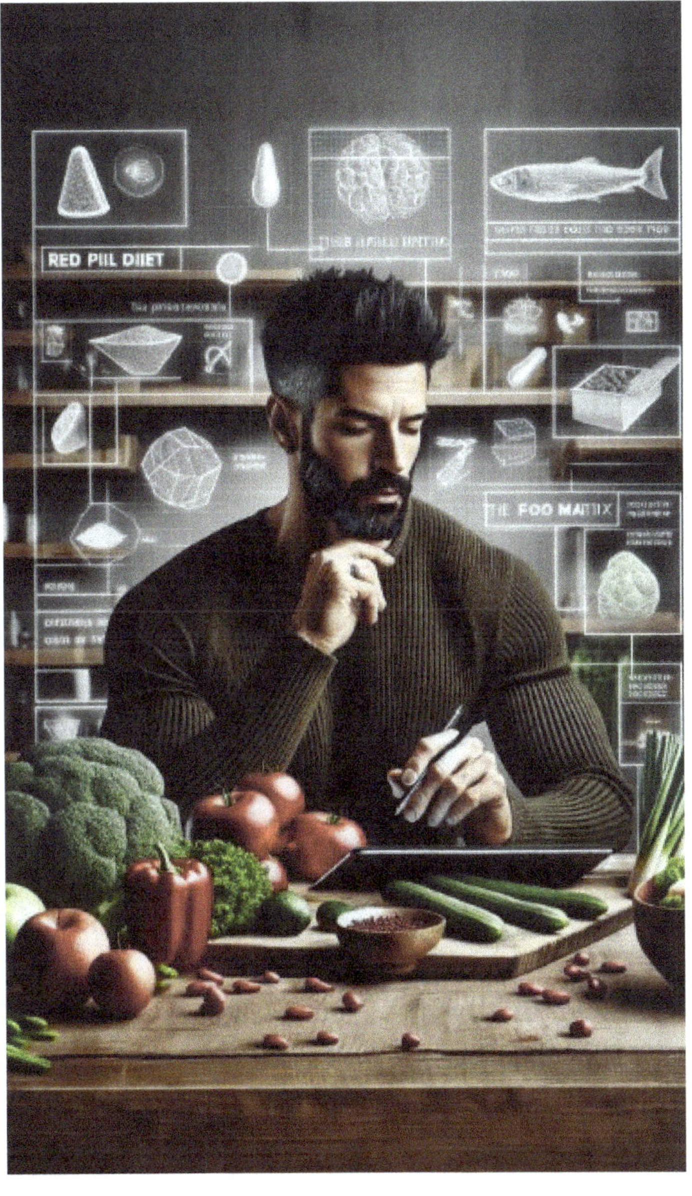

• Creating Your Custom Diet Plan: A Step-by-Step Guide

Crafting a diet that resonates with our unique lifestyle and health goals is paramount; as a health enthusiast, I've navigated through the maze of trendy diets and nutritional misinformation, finding solace in strategies that foster physical health and complete well-being.

Here's my roadmap to developing a diet that's as unique as I am:

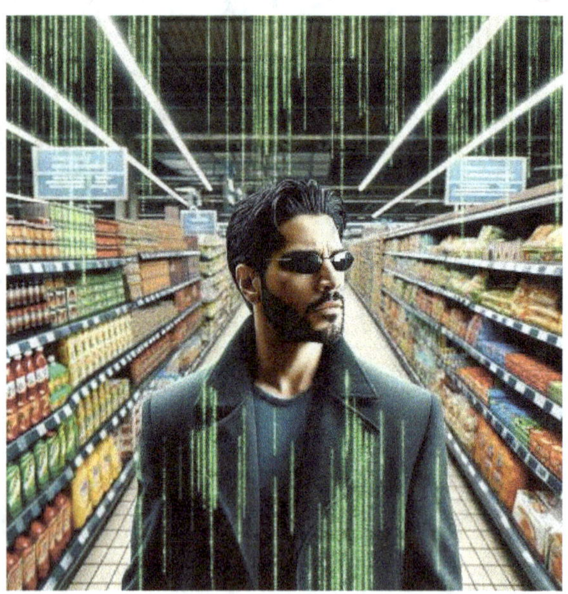

The Red Pill Diet

1. **Self-Reflection on Eating Habits:** My journey began with an honest assessment of my eating habits. Understanding my preferences, recognizing portion sizes, and identifying emotional eating triggers laid the groundwork for my personalized nutrition plan.
2. **Goal Setting:** Clarifying my objectives was crucial. Whether enhancing my overall health or focusing on specific wellness goals, having a clear target provided me with the motivation and direction needed to persist.
3. **Seeking Expertise:** Consulting with nutrition experts—registered dietitians and nutritionists—offered me insights tailored to my unique dietary needs, considering any sensitivities or preferences I had.
4. **Nutritional Literacy:** Diving into the world of macronutrients and micronutrients demystified food science for me. Understanding how different nutrients affect my body empowered me to make informed food choices.

5. **Exploring Dietary Patterns:** Realizing there's no universal solution to dieting, I experimented with various eating patterns—Mediterranean, plant-based, low-carb—to discover what best suited my lifestyle and taste buds.
6. **Mastering Meal Prep:** Planning my meals in advance was a game-changer. It kept impulsive eating at bay and ensured I always had nutritious meals ready, making healthy eating a convenient part of my day.
7. **Embracing Mindful Eating:** Integrating mindfulness into my meals transformed my relationship with food. By eating slowly and savoring each bite, I learned to listen to my body's hunger and fullness cues, fostering a balanced and enjoyable eating experience.

By introducing these strategies into the fabric of my daily life, I've crafted a personalized diet that aligns with my quest for holistic well-being. This approach has taught me that the essence of a healthy lifestyle isn't found in restriction but in creating a harmonious balance that nourishes both body and soul.

· Active Engagement: Applying Learnings Through Challenges

In the whirlwind of today's lifestyle, finding a path to holistic well-being amidst a barrage of fast food ads and the latest diet fads feels like an uphill battle. As a health-conscious person navigating this journey, I've come to realize the power of creating my own personalized plan for nourishing my body and mind. Here's a guide I've crafted, blending strategies and personal insights to help fellow wellness-focused individuals forge their path.

1. Mindful Meal Planning: Take on the challenge of planning your meals mindfully. This involves researching nutritious recipes, creating a shopping list with healthy ingredients, and preparing your meals in advance. By consciously selecting your meals, you'll be more aware of the nutritional value and portion sizes, helping you make healthier choices and avoid impulsive, unhealthy eating.

2. Mindful Eating Journal: Keep a journal dedicated to mindful eating. Document your thoughts and feelings before, during, and after each meal. Reflect on how the food makes you feel physically and emotionally. This practice will help you identify any patterns or triggers that drive unhealthy eating habits, enabling you to make more informed decisions in the future.

3. Smartphone Detox: Challenge yourself to disconnect from your smartphone during meals. This activity encourages you to focus on the present moment and fully savor your food, rather than mindlessly scrolling through social media or watching videos. By eliminating distractions, you can better tune in to your body's hunger and fullness cues, leading to improved portion control and overall eating satisfaction.

4. Mindful Cooking Classes: Engage in cooking classes or workshops that focus on mindful cooking. Learn techniques to prepare nutritious meals while maintaining mindfulness throughout the process. This activity not only enhances your culinary skills but also deepens your understanding of ingredients, their nutritional benefits, and the importance of mindful food preparation.

5. Group Mindful Eating Challenges: Form a support group with fellowwellness seekers on a similar weight loss and nutrition journey. Set weekly or monthly mindful eating challenges together, such as trying new healthy recipes, exploring different cuisines, or experimenting with mindful snacking strategies. This collaborative approach fosters accountability, motivation, and a sense of community, making the weight loss journey more enjoyable and sustainable.

6. Broaden Your Impact by sharing Your Wellness Journey: Embracing the journey toward holistic well-being transcends personal boundaries when you start to share your discoveries and progress. My own path, richly paved with insights from what I've fondly termed the "Mexican Diet," mirrors this belief. This diet, a personal adaptation of the "Red Pill Diet," marries the vibrancy of Healthy Mexican Food with the principles of OMAD (One Meal A Day) and longevity practices. Over seven years, my commitment has evolved through four major iterations, each meticulously documented and shared as engaging infographics.

The Red Pill Diet

But my sharing doesn't stop at mere documentation. By capturing the essence of my journey through photos and videos, I've transformed my personal quest into a narrative that resonates with family, friends, and a broader online community. This digital diary chronicles my evolution and positions me as a dedicated advocate of a lifestyle that champions mindful nutrition and the joy of sharing.

The act of sharing extends beyond simple communication; it's an invitation to inspire and be inspired, creating a ripple effect of wellness advocacy. As I continue to refine and live out the principles of my Red Pill Diet, a.k.a. "The Mexican Diet," the joy of sharing these findings and witnessing their impact on others reaffirms my role as an enthusiast and a knowledgeable guide in mindful eating and living.

Through these strategies, I've woven mindfulness into the fabric of my daily eating habits, stepping away from the noise and into a space where I can nourish my body and soul with intention. It's a testament to the idea that holistic well-being is not a destination but a journey—one that is enriched with every mindful bite.

Beyond the Rabbit Hole: Unveiling the Red Pill Diet within the Food Matrix.

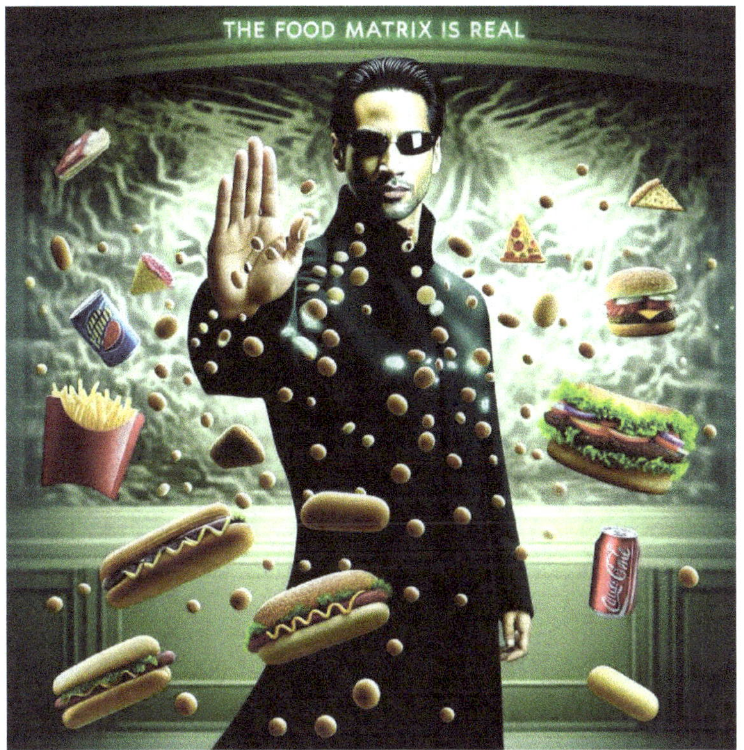

• Empowering Choices: The Power of Awareness and Decision-Making

In the journey toward holistic well-being, navigating the endless sea of dietary advice and wellness trends can feel insurmountable. I've walked this path, grappling with the barrage of information on what to eat, how to exercise, and the endless cycle of diet trends that promise quick results but rarely deliver. This overwhelming flood of advice often leads to confusion, fostering unhealthy habits and efforts at wellness that don't last.

Recognizing our decisions and their effects on our health is the first step toward enduring wellness. In my experience, mindful eating has illuminated this path. It's about tuning into the signals my body sends about hunger and fullness, truly experiencing the flavors and textures of my food, and finding joy in each meal. This approach has deepened my connection with my body, allowing me to hear what it truly needs and fostering a healthier relationship with food.

The critical role of informed decision-making in this process cannot be understated. Amidst the noise, finding reliable, evidence-based information is key. I've learned the importance of understanding nutrition at a deeper level— getting to grips with macronutrients and micronutrients and becoming proficient at interpreting food labels. This knowledge has empowered me to make choices that align with my goals and values, steering clear of fleeting trends and focusing on what truly benefits my health.

Equally, understanding the food industry's influence and marketing strategies has been enlightening. Recognizing the processing behind foods, the ingredients used, and their long-term impacts on health enables me to choose alternatives that not only serve my body better but also promote sustainable practices.

However, this awareness and informed decision-making extend beyond personal health. They're about contributing to a larger ecosystem, supporting whole, unprocessed foods, local farmers, and sustainable agriculture, thus nurturing a healthier planet.

Embarking on this path of mindfulness, education, and conscious choice, I've embraced a lifestyle that supports not just my physical health but my overall well-being. It's a testament to the power of taking control of our dietary choices, armed with knowledge and a commitment to sustainability.

One Red Pill Diet a Day: Sustaining Mindful Eating Practices for Lifelong Health and Happiness

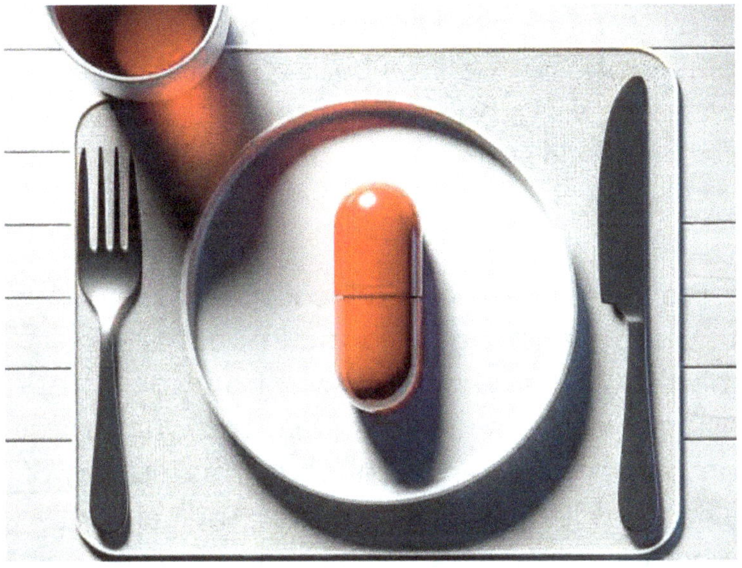

The Red Pill Diet

Mindful eating isn't merely a diet; it's a way of life. It's about engaging fully with eating, about transforming each meal into a moment of clarity and appreciation. In these moments, I've learned to slow down, savor every flavor, and listen genuinely to my body's needs. This practice has unveiled a path to sustainable wellness, a method to counteract the fast-paced chaos surrounding us.

Mindfulness has been my compass. It's led me to understand the profound impact of each food choice, guiding me away from the empty allure of processed fare toward the wholesome embrace of nutrient-rich foods. This journey of awareness is about recognizing the value of what we feed our bodies and making choices that uplift and sustain us, not just in the moment but for the long haul.

Self-compassion has been my sanctuary. In moments of temptation or deviation from my wellness path, I've learned the power of kindness toward myself. Rather than a failure, each stumble has become a step toward deeper understanding and resilience. This gentle, forgiving approach has empowered me to maintain my course toward wellness, even in the face of obstacles.

Consistency, then, is the bridge to lasting transformation. It's not about fleeting commitments or temporary changes but about weaving mindful eating into the very fabric of daily life. This steadfast dedication to mindfulness and self-compassion has reshaped my eating habits and my entire approach to health and happiness.

Setting Realistic Goals

Understanding the importance of achievable targets, I've learned to tailor my health aspirations to fit my unique life context. This chapter of my journey is about guiding you through setting practical, personalized goals in nutrition and wellness, steering clear of the confusion that often shadows our path to a healthier self.

Discerning the valuable from the vacuous is key amid the flood of nutritional advice. I've aimed to cut through the noise, focusing on evidence-based insights that align with my personal health objectives. Setting clear, attainable goals makes the path to well-being less daunting and more structured.

Starting with Self-Assessment: The first step was looking honestly at my dietary habits and overall health. This introspection helped me pinpoint where I stood and where I wanted to head, serving as a compass for my nutritional voyage. It's about knowing your baseline to track your growth and celebrate your progress.

Crafting Specific, Measurable Goals: I veered away from vague ambitions like "eat healthier" toward more tangible, measurable objectives. Small, incremental goals became my milestones, such as incorporating more greens into each meal or reducing processed sugar intake. These specific targets made the journey feel more manageable and rewarding.

Embracing Lifestyle-Compatible Objectives: Acknowledging my routines, responsibilities, and preferences meant setting goals that realistically fit into my life. This approach prevented the disillusionment that often accompanies grand, impractical ambitions, making my wellness path sustainable and enjoyable.

Evolving with Regular Reassessment: As my journey unfolded, so did my understanding of what wellness meant. Continuously reassessing and refining my goals ensured they remained aligned with my evolving needs and insights, keeping me engaged and motivated.

This quest for holistic well-being, grounded in realistic, personalized goals, has illuminated the importance of a mindful, informed approach to nutrition. By prioritizing what truly nourishes us, we pave the way for lasting health and happiness. Let's embark on this path together, embracing the challenges and triumphs that lie ahead, ever mindful not to fall prey to the allure of quick fixes but instead cultivate a deep, nourishing relationship with the food that sustains us.

Creating a Supportive Environment

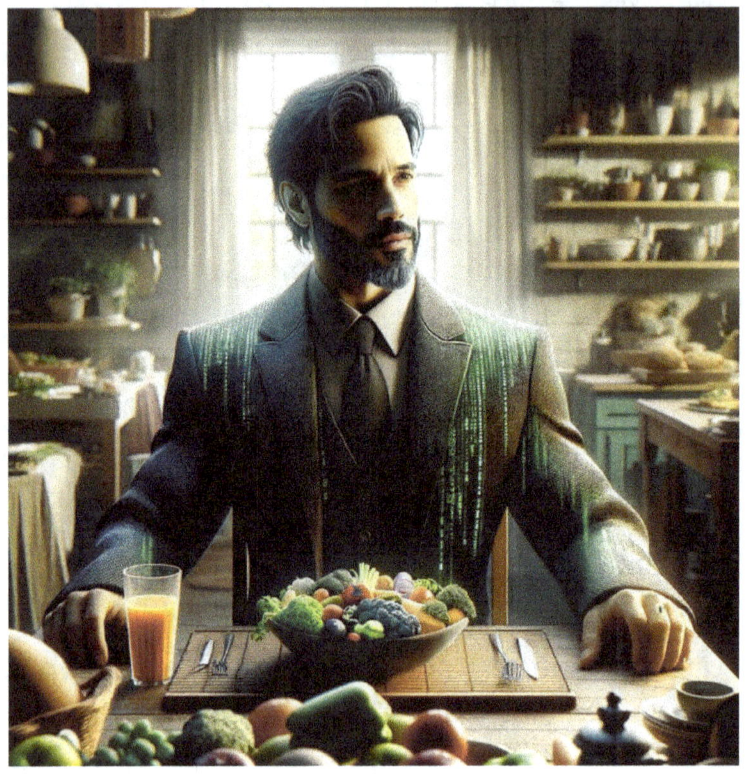

I've realized the profound impact my surroundings have on my dietary choices. This personal journey has taught me that cultivating a supportive environment is beneficial and essential for nurturing healthy eating habits. Here, I share insights and strategies that have guided me in shaping a space that champions nutritious eating and bolsters my commitment to a healthier lifestyle.

Stocking Up on Nutritious Foods:

My first step was to transform my pantry. I made it a haven for nutrient-rich foods, stocking up on fresh fruits, vegetables, whole grains, lean proteins, and healthy fats. This simple act of choosing what fills my shelves has been pivotal. It means the convenience of reaching for something wholesome is always within arm's reach, steering me away from the lure of processed snacks and sugary treats.

Kitchen Organization for Mindful Eating:

Rearranging my kitchen to highlight healthy options became a game-changer. I naturally gravitated toward better choices by positioning nutritious snacks at eye level and tucking away less healthy items. Embracing tools like food storage containers and portion control aids further reinforced this supportive ecosystem, making mindful eating an effortless part of my routine.

Building a Community of Wellness Seekers:

Embarking on this journey alongside others zealously for healthy living has amplified my resolve. Whether through local nutrition groups or vibrant online communities, connecting with individuals on similar paths has enriched my experience with shared wisdom, motivation, and a sense of accountability.

Creating a Mindful Dining Space:

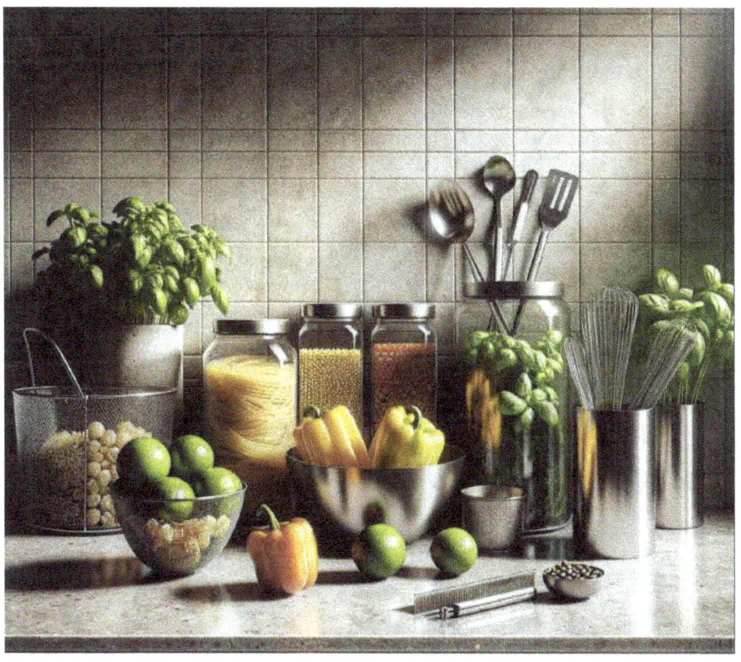

I've learned that the ambiance in which we eat
profoundly affects our meal choices and
enjoyment. Dining in a serene, distraction-free
setting allows me to fully engage with the act
of eating, enhancing my appreciation for
flavors and promoting a more mindful
relationship with food. Introducing elements
of nature and ensuring ample natural light in
my dining area have made mealtimes more
tranquil and satisfying.

Sustaining Healthy Habits for Life

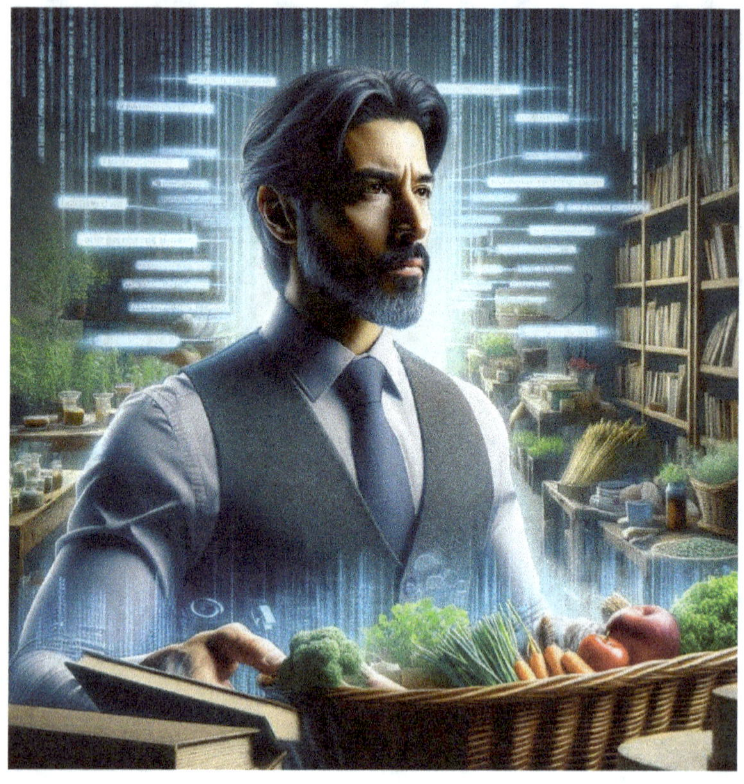

The Red Pill Diet

In the quest for holistic well-being, embracing the nuanced journey of nutrition has become a central theme of my life. Here, I share a path carved through personal experience and learning, aiming to inspire fellow wellness seekers to cultivate lifelong healthy habits. This guide reflects a blend of dedication, curiosity, and resilience in navigating the complex world of nutrition.

Embracing Nutritional Wisdom: My adventure began with a deep dive into the world of nutrition. I sought to unravel the mysteries of macronutrients and micronutrients, understanding their pivotal roles in our health. This journey of knowledge wasn't just about accumulating facts but about equipping myself to make enlightened choices for my well-being.

Questioning the Nutritional Quagmire: I learned early on the importance of questioning the myriad of dietary advice that floods our lives. Distinguishing between scientifically backed insights and pervasive myths became my mantra. This discernment has been crucial in filtering the noise and focusing on what truly benefits my health.

The Red Pill Diet

Personalizing My Plate: Adopting healthy eating habits was more than a decision; it was a commitment to myself. From mindful meal planning that reflects my unique lifestyle to embracing portion control without compromising on satisfaction, I tailored my nutritional practices to be both joyous and sustainable.

Exploring the Mind-Food Connection: The journey also led me to explore the emotional landscapes of eating. Understanding emotional eating triggers and fostering a positive relationship with food became pillars of my approach. It's about nurturing the body and mind, recognizing that our thoughts and emotions play a significant role in our dietary choices.

Cultivating Community Support: I've found solace and strength in a community of health-conscious peers. Through forums, workshops, and local wellness groups, the exchange of stories and strategies has been both uplifting and enlightening. This sense of belonging and mutual encouragement has been a cornerstone of my journey.

Embracing Dietary Exploration: Creating a diet that reflects my unique needs and preferences was a journey of exploration. It required an open mind, patience, and a willingness to experiment. Through trial and error, I discovered the balance of foods that made me feel my best. This exploration taught me that nutritional well-being isn't about rigidly following a prescribed set of rules but about finding joy and balance in the foods that serve my body and spirit.

The Culmination of Personal Clarity: This 'aha moment'—the realization that my path to wellness is mine to define—was transformative. It's not merely about what I eat but how I connect with my food, understanding its impact on my body and how it aligns with my values and lifestyle. This personal clarity has been the key to developing a sustainable approach to eating that celebrates my individuality and supports my journey towards a vibrant, nourished life.

Beyond the Matrix:
A New Vision for Nutritional Empowerment

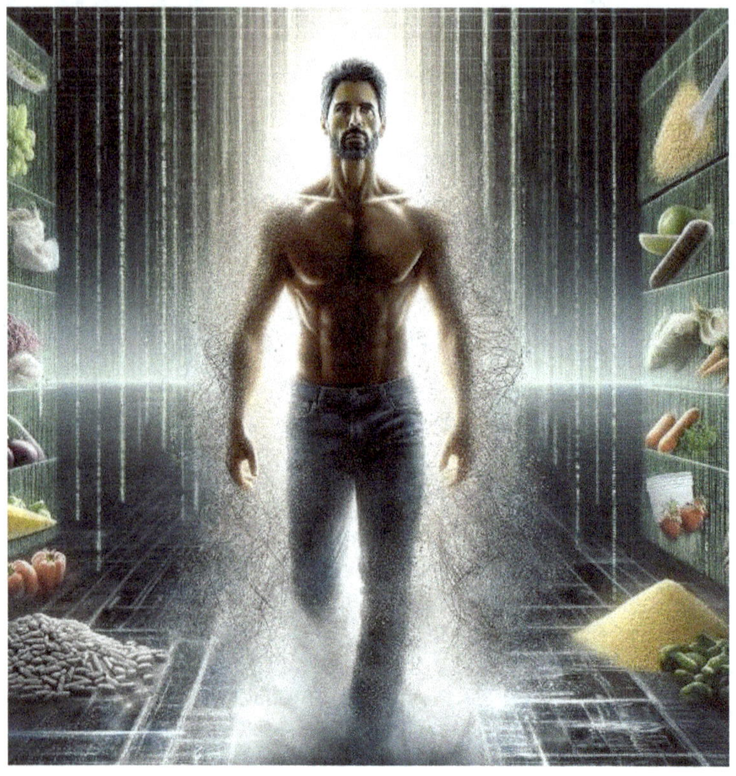

As we conclude our insightful journey through The Food Matrix, let's welcome the end of our voyage with a refreshed outlook. This concluding chapter acts as a mirror to our experiences and a light guiding us onwards., encapsulating the essence of our collective epiphanies and the profound shifts in our understanding of nutrition and health.

We began entangled within The Food Matrix, a complex web spun from the threads of misinformation and commercial interests, which often obscured the path to true nutritional well-being. Through our shared odyssey, we've unraveled these intricacies, armed with the knowledge and insight to distinguish between the fleeting allure of processed conveniences and the enduring vitality offered by whole, unadulterated foods. Our journey illuminated the critical importance of questioning, learning, and adapting—a perpetual cycle of enlightenment that challenges us to refine our dietary choices in alignment with evolving scientific insights and our body's innate wisdom.

The Red Pill Diet

This narrative invites you to continue the voyage beyond the pages, encouraging an ongoing commitment to nutritional discovery and self-empowerment. As we step forth, let's carry the torch of curiosity, illuminating our path toward a life unshackled from The Food Matrix. This is not an end but a beginning—a call to action for all who seek to nourish not just the body but the soul in a world brimming with both challenges and opportunities for growth.

Embrace this journey as your own, for every small step toward understanding and implementing the principles of true nutrition is a leap toward freedom, vitality, and well-being. Together, let's forge ahead, inspired and unyielding, as we continue to uncover the truths that empower us to live our healthiest lives, unbound by The Food Matrix.

Dietary Liberation:
A Manifesto for Personalized Nutrition

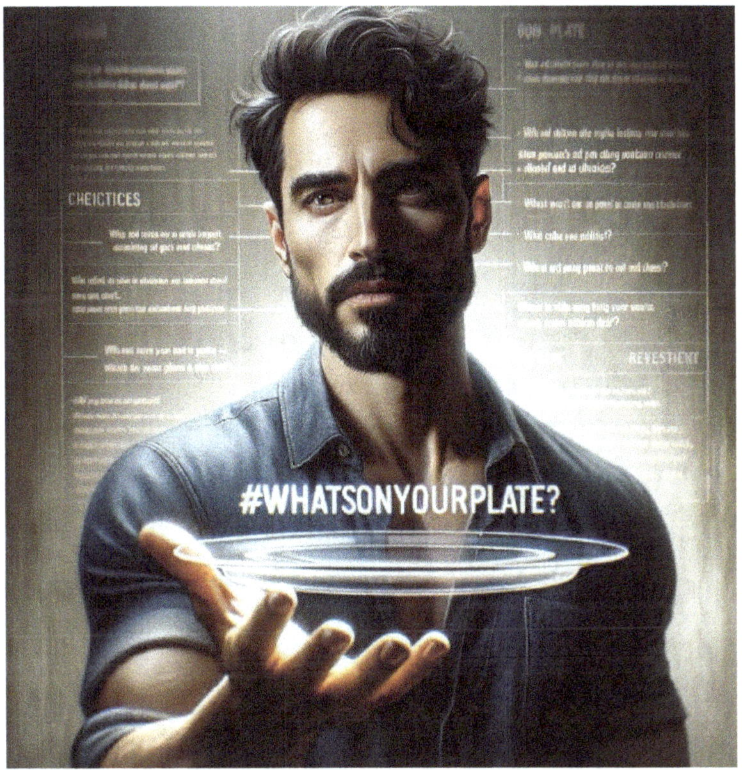

The Red Pill Diet

My vision is clear and resolute: to forge a guide that empowers humanity to break away from the confining narratives of "the Food Matrix," narratives crafted and perpetuated by the food companies that have long dictated our choices. This guide, "The Red Pill Diet," is not just a collection of dietary recommendations— it's a manifesto for liberation from the one-size-fits-all dieting dogma.

I look to a future where the lexicon of "the Food Matrix," "the Blue Pill Diet," and "the Red Pill Diet" becomes ingrained in our daily conversations. These terms will not just be buzzwords but symbols of a cultural shift towards nutritional enlightenment and autonomy. They will represent a collective awakening to the importance of bespoke diets that celebrate our unique needs and preferences.

In this future, the act of sharing one's "Red Pill Diet" is a celebration of individuality, a discussion that goes beyond mere food preferences to embody a statement of self-identity and personal philosophy. It's a world where our diets are as distinctive as our fingerprints, proudly shared and respected as expressions of our singularity.

Appendix

ChatGPT Book Companion

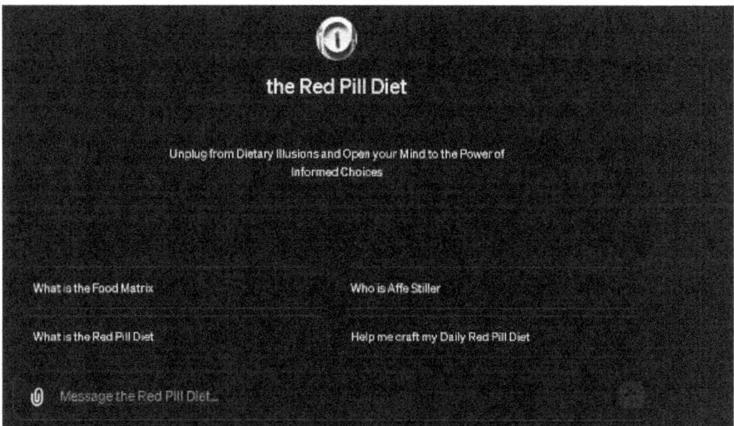

Introducing a "ChatGPT Book Companion" represents a groundbreaking innovation in the ever-evolving world of health and longevity. This digital companion goes beyond the traditional use of AI for answering questions, offering a wealth of original applications designed to enhance your journey toward a healthier, longer life. Here's a list of 10 original uses and applications that showcase its versatility:

The Red Pill Diet

1. **Personalized Nutrition Plans:** Tailor your diet to your specific health goals, lifestyle, and preferences, with customized meal plans and nutritional advice.
2. **Interactive Recipe Modification:** Adapt recipes on the fly to suit dietary restrictions, allergies, or simply to work with ingredients you have on hand.
3. **Dynamic Fitness Coaching:** Receive guided workout plans and adjustments based on progress, preferences, and performance feedback.
4. Sleep Optimization Strategies: Get personalized recommendations for improving sleep quality and duration, crucial for overall health and longevity.
5. **Stress Reduction Techniques:** Learn and apply mindfulness exercises, breathing techniques, and other strategies to reduce stress and enhance well-being.
6. **Educational Explorations:** Deep dive into the science of longevity, with explanations, summaries, and discussions on the latest research and theories.

7. **Health Tracking and Analysis:** Create a log of your daily habits, from diet to exercise to sleep, and receive analyses and recommendations for improvement.

8. **Community Connection:** Engage with a community of like-minded individuals, share experiences, and find motivation and support.

9. **Virtual Health Challenges:** Participate in virtual challenges designed to improve health and habits, with progress tracking and rewards for achievements.

10. **Mindfulness and Meditation Guides:** Access guided meditation sessions and mindfulness exercises tailored to your needs and preferences, enhancing mental and emotional health.

This ChatGPT Book Companion brings the convenience of ubiquity, allowing you to carry a personal coach in your pocket, accessible anytime, anywhere. Its capabilities are not just limited to answering questions but extend to creating a dynamic, interactive learning and living experience. Whether you're looking to refine your diet, enhance your physical fitness, or deepen your understanding of longevity practices, this tool is designed to support you every step of the way.

The Red Pill Diet

Go to whatisthefoodmatrix.com or scan the QR code down below and give it a try with these conversation starters:

- "What's a simple recipe I can start with for a plant-based diet?"
- "Show me a 15-minute workout routine I can do at home."
- "How can I improve my sleep quality starting tonight?"
- "Teach me a five-minute mindfulness exercise to reduce stress."

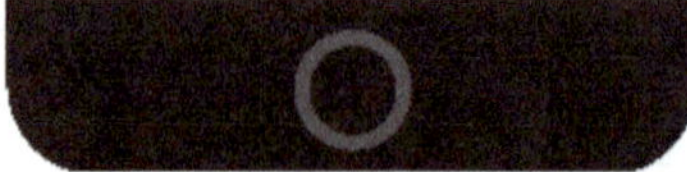

Unlock the full potential of your ChatGPT companion for free; just ensure you're subscribed to ChatGPT Plus for uninterrupted, premium access.

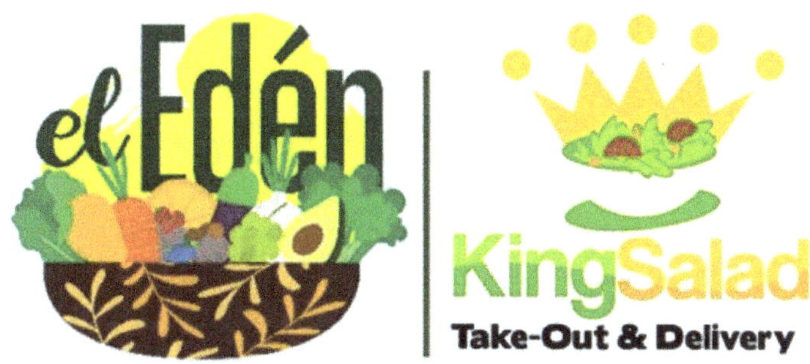

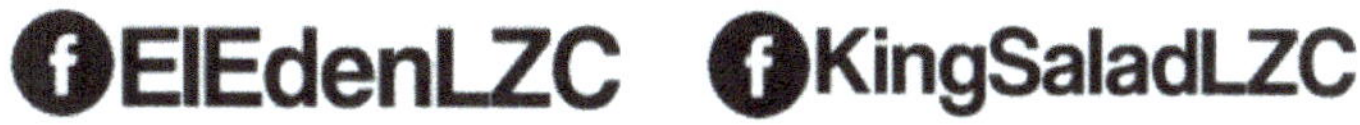

At the heart of this narrative is "El Eden," a sanctuary of healthful cuisine crafted by Affe Stiller and his partner, Euridice.

Born amidst the global pause of the pandemic, "El Eden" was their beacon to the community, offering solace through nutrition in Mexico. The kitchen became a canvas for their creativity, blending the guiding principles of whole plant-based nutrition with Euridice's culinary artistry.

Together, they reimagined traditional Mexican dishes into vegan masterpieces alongside Euridice's innovative creations, making "El Eden" a testament to the power of plant-based healing.

Their experience has been profound. Countless individuals have reported immediate positive shifts, with many returning to normal biometric levels swiftly. Those who embraced the regimen for six months or more often appeared five to ten years younger, all thanks to the transformative power of plant-based Mexican cuisine.

Appendix 2

Affe Stiller´s Red Pill Diet

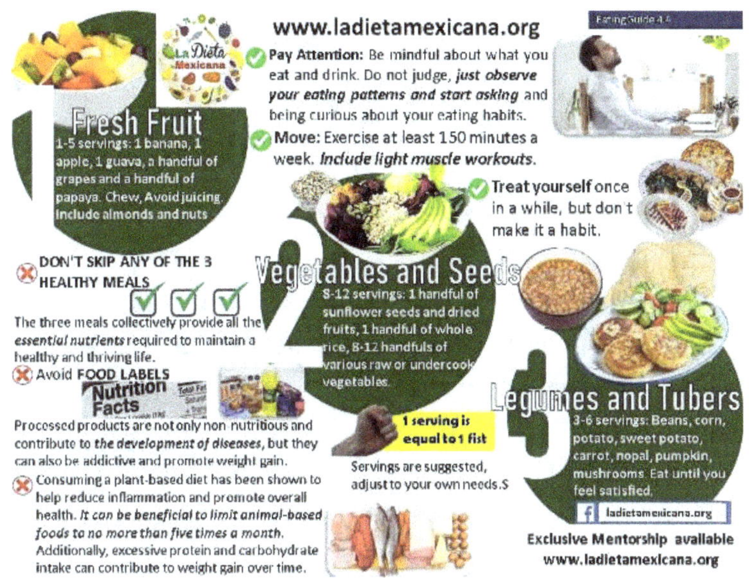

themexicandiet.com/the-mexican-diet

La Dieta Mexicana de la Longevidad

Affe Stiller, a luminary in the journey toward nutritional enlightenment, offers a vision that transcends the conventional.

His approach to "The Mexican Longevity Diet" is not merely a temporary regimen but a lifelong commitment to sustainable health.

This ethos embraces a diet enriched daily with a vibrant mosaic of fruits, green vegetables, seeds, grains, nuts, legumes (including beans, lentils, chickpeas, etc.), and tubers (potatoes, sweet potatoes, chayote), seasoned with herbs and spices tailored to personal tastes.

It's a testament to living in harmony with nature's bounty, ensuring a sustainable and nourishing path for life.

Engaging with Affe Stiller: Topics for Discussion and Collaboration

Affe Stiller is open to sharing his deep well of knowledge and experience through various platforms and mediums. Whether it's a podcast, an interview, a signature engagement, or a speaking event, Affe brings thought-provoking insights and actionable wisdom to every conversation.

Here is a curated list of topics Affe is passionate about and more than happy to explore:

Conscious Eating - How to make mindful food choices that align with the nourishment of body and soul.

Longevity Training - Strategies to live a long, vibrant life through consistent, mindful practices.

The Mexican Diet - Integrating the wisdom of traditional Mexican eating principles for optimal health.

The Red Pill Diet

Mindfulness Coaching - Techniques for staying present and managing daily stress.

Intermittent Fasting - Understanding the benefits and methods of effective fasting.

Meaningful Conversations - Fostering deep, insightful discussions for personal and professional growth.

Motivational Guidance - Finding and pursuing one's personal goals and ambitions.

Purpose Discovery - Helping individuals unearth their life's purpose.

Yoga Mental - Practices to enhance mental flexibility and strength.

Minimalist Living - Simplifying life to focus on what truly matters.

Entrepreneurial Marketing Expertise - Leveraging a rich entrepreneurial journey to create and market unique value propositions.

Affe Stiller is excited to discuss these topics, among others, bringing unique insights and value to your audience. His experiences are not just lessons but transformative tools for those ready to embrace change.

To book Affe Stiller for your next event, visit www.theredpilldiet.ai or scan the QR code below.

The Red Pill Diet Soundtrack

In the journey of unraveling the Food Matrix, music plays a pivotal role, serving as both a muse and a medium for distilling wisdom.

Affe Stiller, in his quest to illuminate the path toward a conscious dietary lifestyle, has meticulously curated a selection of songs that echo the essence of his transformative insights.

These melodies are gathered in the Spotify playlists Azucarniuna and VeloxVeritasMatrix, and also celebrated under the hashtag #matrixsongs on Facebook, capturing the rhythm of awakening and the harmony of enlightenment.

Every song serves as a strand interwoven into the fabric of The Red Pill Diet, providing listeners with an auditory journey through the themes intricately laced within the pages of this book.

Scan the QR code and immerse yourself in the sounds that inspired Affe Stiller to challenge the norms and champion a life unbound by the Food Matrix.

Let this musical journey complement your reading, as you savor another layer of wisdom distilled through melody.

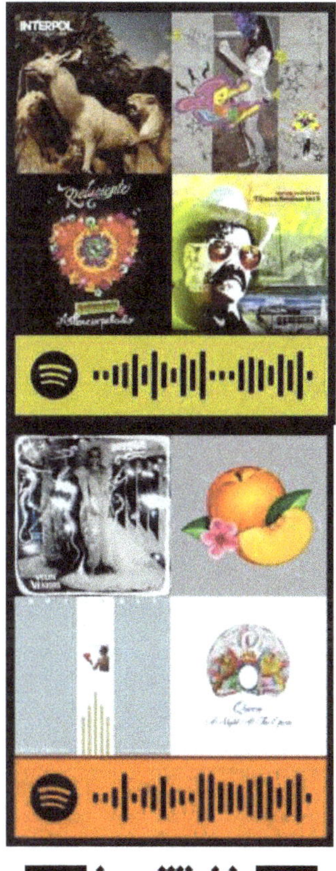

9 7 9 8 3 2 0 4 6 3 1 0 0